THE WISDOM OF JESUS
AND THE YOGA SIDDHAS

by
Marshall Govindan

Babaji's Kriya Yoga and Publications, Inc.
St. Etienne de Bolton, Quebec, Canada

The Wisdom of Jesus and the Yoga Siddhas
by Marshall Govindan

First published in April 2007 by
Babaji's Kriya Yoga and Publications, Inc.
196 Mountain Road, P.O. Box 90,
Eastman, Quebec, Canada J0E 1P0
Telephone: 450-297-0258; 1-888-252-9642; fax: 450-297-3957
· www.babaji.ca · email: info@babaji.ca

Copyright © 2006 by Marshall Govindan
Reprinted or used with the permission of:
Oxford University Press Copyright © 2003: excerpts from *Lost Christianities: The Battles for Scriputre and the Faiths We Never Knew,* by Bart Ehrman. Scribner, an imprint of Simon & Schuster Adult Publishing Group, from *The Five Gospels What did Jesus Really Say?*, by Robert Funk, Roy Hoover and the Jesus Seminar. Copyright © 1993 by Polebridge Press. Harper Collins Publishers, Inc: excerpts from pages 23, 42-43, 45, 50, 65, 77, 116 from *The Gospel of Thomas:The Hidden Sayings of Jesus,* by Marvin Meyer English translation and critical edition of the Coptic text. Copyright © 1992 by Marvin Meyer. Interpretation by Harold Bloom. Copyright © 1992 by Harold Bloom; and pages 36-38 from *The Gospel According to Jesus,* by Stephen Mitchell, reprinted by permission of Harper Collins Publishers Random House, Inc. from *The Gnostic Gospels,* copyright © *1979* by Elaine Pagels.

All rights reserved. No part of this book may be reproduced or utilized in any form or by any means, electronic or mechanical, including photocopying, recording, or by any information storage and retrieval system, without permission in writing from the publisher.

Cover design: Sonia Giguere

Printed and bound in Canada. 100% printed on recycled paper

Babaji's Kriya Yoga and Publications wishes to thank the Société de développement des enterprises culturels du Québec for their financial support in publishing this work.

Care has been taken to trace the ownership of any copyright material contained in this text. The publishers welcome any information that will enable them to rectify in subsequent editions, any incorrect or omitted reference or credit.

Library and Archives Canada Cataloguing in Publication

Govindan, Marshall
    The Wisdom of Jesus and the Yoga Siddhas / by Marshall Govindan

Includes bibliographical references.
ISBN 978-1-895383-43-0

        1. Christianity and yoga. 2. Jesus Christ –Teachings – Meditations.
        3. Yoga. I. Title.

BR128.Y63G68 2007   261.2'45   C2006-906957-3

Dedication

To

Father Thomas O. King, S.J.

for sowing the seeds of my interest in the authentic teachings of Jesus during my first year as a student at Georgetown University

Acknowledgements

I am grateful to many students and friends for their support in conducting the research over the past six years, resulting in this publication. In particular Dr. Georg Feuerstein Ph.D., who co-founded with me the Yoga Siddha Research Project in 2000. Also, Joan Ruvinsky, Tom Motz, Markus Doll, Kim Houtz, George Turpin, Chris Jalowy, Subashini Yalamanchi, Douglas Lawson, Scott Anderson of the Yoga Research and Education Center, and many other friends and students for financial support to this research project. I am grateful to Dr. T.N. Ganapathy Ph.D., its Director and General editor, Ph.D. and Dr. KR Arumugam Ph.D., his deputy, S.N. Kandaswamy, T.V. Venkateswaran, and Dr. Siddhalingaiah Ph.D., for their scholarship and dedicated service to this project, which has so far produced six major publications.

I would like to thank above all, my wife, Durga Jan Ahlund, for her review of each draft of this book, and for her helpful and insightful comments, as well as her constant support and love.

Special thanks also to Ramanathan Iyer, Reverend Fred Anderson, Carl Ahlund and David Frawley for many helpful suggestions on the manuscript of this book.

I would like to thank Don Wagner for his efforts in copy editing this book, and the other reviewers for their comments and encouragement.

Special thanks to Sonia Giguere for the graphic layout of this book, and for the cover design.

I am grateful to the late Yogi S.A.A. Ramaiah, who, beginning in 1970, inspired me to study the works of the Yoga Siddhas, and who trained me in their hidden teachings.

Marshall Govindan
February 16, 2007 (Mahashivratri)

Contents

Prologue by the author   8

Introduction
    Questions   21
    Remarkable Similarities   24
    Why Should Christian Study Yoga?   30
    The Objectives of This Book   32

Chapter 1 Modern Historical Research of Jesus and Early Christianity   35
    The Development of the Seven Pillars of Modern Historical Biblical Research   37
    Methodology and Findings of Modern Critical Biblical Scholars   39
    Were the Gospels Inerrant and Inspired by God?   43
    Two Portraits of Jesus: the Map of Relationships Between the Gospels   45
    Rules of Written Evidence   48
    The Oral Tradition Prior to the Gospels and the Rules of Oral Evidence   51
    The Distinctive Voice of Jesus   53
    The Unassertive Sage   54

Chapter 2 The Paradoxical Teachings of the God-men   56
    The Problem of Paradox   57
    What Did Jesus Really Do According to Modern Historical Research?   58
    What is Yoga?   59
    Yoga as a Philosophy   60
    Who Are the Yoga Siddhas?   63
    What is the Literature of the Yoga Siddhas?   70
    Similarities Between Jesus and the Yoga Siddhas and Their Teachings   74
    Was Jesus a Guru?   89
    Devotees Versus Disciples   94

Are There Any Differences Between Jesus and the Yoga Siddhas?	95
Was Jesus a Yoga Siddhas?	97

Chapter 3 Gospel of Thomas: A Gnostic Text? — 98
History and Distinctiveness of the Gospel of Thomas	99
The Gospel of Thomas: A Gnostic Text?	101
The Kingdom of Heaven is Already Here	103
The Hidden, Gnostic Heart of the Gospel of Thomas: Jesus as Initiator of His Most Worthy Disciples into Esoteric Knowledge: Gnosis	106
Discounting the Value of Prophecy and its Fulfillment for our Freedom	108
Who Am I?	109
On Entering into the Kingdom of Heaven	111
Was Jesus a Gnostic?	112
How is One to Realize the Gnosis, the Saving Knowledge	114

Chapter 4 Early Christianity: the Formation of the Church and its Dogma — 117
The Dead Sea Scrolls and the Essenes	117
Early Christian Historical Sources	119
Paulism	120
Early Doctrinal Issues	122
Docetism	123
Ebionitism	123
Marcionites	124
The Gnostics	125
The Proto-Orthodox	127
The Cultural and Political Factors Which Favored the Proto-Orthodox	131
The Rule of Faith and Creeds	134
The Gospel of John Versus the Gospels of Thomas, Matthew, Mark and Luke	135
The Formation of the Proto-Ortodox New Testament	137
Constantine and the Ecumenical Council of Nicaea	140

Chapter 5 What Did Jesus Really Say? — 142
Reversing Natural Human Inclinations	143
The Kingdom of Heaven	145
On Entering into the Kingdom of Heaven	147
Why Should Jesus Say that Those Who are Poor, Hungry, Suffering and Persecuted are Blessed?	150
On Purity	151
On Worry, and Being Present	152
On Aspiration	154
Showing the Path to Others	156
The Lord's Prayer	159
God's Unconditional Love	160
Forgiveness of Sins and the Karmic Consequences of our Actions	164

Hidden Treasure	167
The Good Samaritan	168

Chapter 6 What Did Jesus Not Say? 170
Gospel of John	171
The "I am" Sayings	173
The Farewell Prayer	175
The End of the World	176
Jesus' Dying Words	177
At the Tomb	178
Doubting Thomas	178
The Familiar Tenets of Christianity Cannot Be Traced to Jesus Himself	178
Christianity Was Founded by Paul	181
Consequences of Christianity's Replacing the Teachings of Jesus	182

Conclusion and Recommendations 184

Notes 188

Bibliographic References 193

Glossary 197

Appendix A: Index of Red and Pink letter sayings from Jesus Seminar 206

Prologue by the Author

The origin of this book lies in my experience and education as a Christian during my early years, and in my search for the spiritual teachings of Jesus. Anyone making an historical, philosophical or scientific enquiry, brings much which is personal to the task. It will be helpful, therefore, for the reader to know where "I am coming from." I owe to my parents, Jane and Harry, a deep debt of gratitude for having shared with me their faith in Jesus Christ during the first eighteen years of my life. From 1953 to 1967, my mother was a Sunday school teacher and superintendent in the local Lutheran Church on Sepulveda Boulevard in Westchester, California, two miles north of the Los Angeles International Airport. My father served it in various capacities, including Treasurer. My earliest memories include ones involving religious services in the old sanctuary, particularly at Easter and Christmas, when the special decorations and fervor of the members of the congregation, friends of our family, filled me with love and joy. That "God is love" was made manifest in the warm community of this church. I delighted in singing hymns and found inspiration in the sermons of Pastor Olsen and later Pastor Anderson. My friends were Christians and I enjoyed periodic "Christian Youth" rallies and field trips to churches in far off places like Phoenix, Arizona.

When I was twelve years old I attended a Billy Graham rally with a hundred thousand other persons at the Los Angeles Coliseum. I was overwhelmed by its intensity, and when Billy Graham called upon us to come down to the stage and declare our commitment to Jesus Christ, I responded, and went. I accepted Jesus Christ as my Lord and Savior. For many months thereafter I studied the lessons which his organization sent to me in the mail. I also began to dream of one day becoming a Christian missionary in Africa.

But there were questions, and I was not satisfied. I recall that even when I was about seven years old, I asked Pastor Olsen: "What happens to good people who are not Christians after they die? Do they go to heaven or hell?" This question arose in my mind because my father had recently begun to share his passion for stamp collecting with me. He had given me my first stamp collection, including many stamps from many foreign countries, including many British and French colonies in Africa, the South Pacific and Southeast Asia. I became aware that there were many different cultures and they were not like mine. Pastor Olsen's reply surprised me: "They go to hell," he said. Somewhere from within myself, however, I heard myself quietly saying: "This cannot be true. God loves everyone. He would not send good persons to hell just because they were not Christian!"

When I was thirteen I attended Catechism classes at the Lutheran Church, conducted by Pastor Anderson, and became more familiar with the doctrines of our faith. These classes awoke within me many questions. I recall asking Pastor Anderson what "heaven" was like. He replied that he could not say, because it was not described in the Bible. I asked him "what is sin." His answer was much more satisfying: "Ignorance of the presence of God." But could I know the presence of God? Could I not find God, if He exists in the world? I was left dissatisfied and resolved to begin my search for a way to know God.

When I was fifteen years old I attended a "Human Encounter Session" at the local Y.M.C.A., a half mile down the road from Westchester Lutheran Church. For two full days, about sixty of my classmates from high school sat in a circle and shared our concerns about life. We talked and listened to one another for hours. A Y.M.C.A. counselor gently moderated the discussions, giving everyone an opportunity to share their heartfelt insights and questions. Near the end of the second day, the discussion died down. No one had anything more to say. We seemed to have collectively reached a place of rest. Suddenly, I had my first spiritual experience. I transcended my ordinary mental state and entered into a state of quiet ecstasy. I realized that there was only one Being in the room who was speaking earnestly through all of us, guiding us back to the realization of our true identity, beyond names and forms. This Being permeated everything, and was totally loving and benevolent. I was transfixed by the experience, and for days afterwards enjoyed an altered state of consciousness wherein I felt the oneness of everything. It was truer than anything that I had ever experienced before. Though I could not describe it, I knew that "It" or "That," which I had perceived as my Self, and as the Reality behind everything was the Source of everything. Gradually, however, this state went away. It left me with the deepest longing to find it again. I began to read books which would help me to find it again: those of Alan Watts, the American Zen Buddhist practitioner, whose contemporary expressions reminded me of "That," which I had experienced. I also began to practice meditation, as suggested by Alan Watts' books, seeking to quiet the mind, watching the breath, sitting still with my back straight, in the backyard of my parents' home.

At the same time, I took my high school studies seriously. I was inspired by John F. Kennedy's challenge: "Ask not what your country can do for you. Ask what you can do for your country." I enjoyed reading about current events, particularly about all of the colonies in Africa, which were becoming independent countries during those years, including the Belgian Congo. So, in 1963, when I was fifteen years old I traveled alone by Greyhound Bus to Washington, D.C. to visit a school that I had read about: The School of Foreign Service at Georgetown University. While in Washington, D.C. I visited the Congress, the White House, the Smithsonian and the Lincoln and Jefferson Memorials, and this strengthened my resolve to dedicate my life to public service. So, by the time I was sixteen years old I had decided to seek a career in the U.S. Foreign Service, as a diplomat, and to apply to Georgetown University. When I was accepted by Georgetown two years later, I was overjoyed, for I had a clear vision of my life's work.

When, at the end of the summer of 1966, I arrived at Georgetown University, and found my room in the New North Dormitory, one of the first persons I met was Father Thomas O. King, S.J. He lived in a small room, not much bigger than the room I shared with my roommate, on the same hallway where thirty of us freshman lived. He was the "supervisor" and spiritual counselor for those who were assigned to a room on this hallway. As Georgetown University was the oldest Catholic university in North America, I imagine that at one time, the duties of such "supervisors" were much more invasive of the personal space and freedom of students. Father King, then in his mid-forties, looked like an ascetic: thin, pale, gentle and mild, with large glowing eyes. I learned from another student that he was the resident "demonologist" of Georgetown, and that a few years before he had successfully exorcised a young patient at Georgetown University Hospital's psychiatric ward. I was told that the psychiatrists had tried unsuccessfully to cure this young patient, and in desperation requested the Church to attempt a "spiritual intervention." Over a long period, Father King succeeded in learning the names of thirteen demons which, so the story went, inhabited this young man. Having at last identified them by name, Father King was then able to perform the medieval rite of exorcism, calling forth and banishing these demons in name of "our Lord Jesus Christ." In doing this, the demons reportedly attempted to possess Father King and in the ensuing struggle, Father King nearly died. However, because of his love for Jesus Christ, the demons not only left the young man, but also failed to overcome Father King. This dramatic tale kept us in awe of Father King, and we generally gave him lots of space. He was there for us, if we needed him, but he rarely intervened in our lives, unless someone was making too much noise late at night, after drinking a bit too much at one of the local pubs. A few years later, another Georgetown student, Peter Blattie, wrote the book, *The Exorcist*, which Hollywood then made into a film at Georgetown, a couple of blocks away.

Georgetown was a Catholic institution in transition during the 1960's. Pope John XXIII's Vatican II Council sent waves of reform throughout the Church. Mass was conducted every morning in Dahlgren Chapel, right next to our dormitory, but it was no longer conducted in Latin. As students we were still required to wear a suit or sports jacket and tie to class and attend classes related to religion. While most of the students were the scions of America's Catholic elite, also attending were the sons and daughters of many foreign diplomats assigned to Washington, D.C. and a few others of us who were not Catholic. I attended one religion class called "Christian marriage," taught by Father Bradley, who taught from the Papal Encyclical on this subject. It was of course at variance with the "sexual revolution" going on around us, with the introduction of the birth control "pill." While many of our professors were Jesuit priests, some were Arab scholars, ex-diplomats, and German scholars of medieval history. Classical studies were giving way to "liberation theology" and "women's studies."

I felt apart of a new movement in America. Martin Luther King's civil rights movement was all around us, particularly with the eruption of Washington D.C., following his assassination. There was also a small, but growing opposition on campus to the Vietnam War, lead by Father McSorley, who was also making an impression upon me. Father McSorley was a friend and priest to Senator Bobby Kennedy and his family. He took myself and a few other students, with him, to meet the Senator one weekend at his home in Hickory Hill, Virginia. Our student body President was Bill Clinton.

My continuing interest in religion included during my sophomore year, a class in Comparative Religion, study of Huston Smith's book on world religions, regular attendance at the local Anglican Church services, and most importantly, participation in Father King's "Exploration into Spirit" class where we explored the spiritual side of world religions. I was fascinated by the works of Teilhard de Chardin and Thomas Merton, and the realization that behind all of the differing forms of religious expression, there was a formless, inexpressible truth, which mystics throughout the ages had born testimony too. Father King organized weekend retreats for us at a local Jesuit seminary in Maryland, where we were taught how to go deep within ourselves to experience this timeless truth, in silence. I also learned that Father King himself spent many of his weekends in personal retreats with Tibetan lamas. He was, I knew, not your typical Jesuit priest. I felt that "he knew." My confidence in him would prove to be crucial, during a subsequent crisis of faith, two years later, during my senior year.

I had spent my junior year abroad at Fribourg University in Switzerland, a medieval Catholic sort of place, where I studied *"Ethique Sociale"* with a Benedictine scholar, Father Utz, as well as international economics. I was attempting, I believe, to reconcile my interest in public service and my growing interest in spirituality. A growing disenchantment with the former, due to the Viet Nam war, made the latter much more attractive. I felt a need to escape, and did so for a time, by skiing and by traveling to Spain and Morocco, Paris and London. A six month hiatus from student life brought me face to face with the likes of Salvador Dali and members of his entourage in Cadecus, Spain and with many of the "beautiful people" of London and Paris. This short escapade into a rather hedonistic lifestyle came crashing down on me, and I knew I had to return to school in Fribourg, to recuperate from my misadventures and reflect deeply upon the purpose of my life. When I returned, I began to write a novel, based upon my experiences, one, to get it out of my system, and two, to get some perspective on myself.

I returned at the end of the year to my parents' home in California. It was there, just as I was completing work on my novel, when I was introduced to Paramahansa Yogananda and his book, *Autobiography of a Yogi*. John Probe, a friend of my sister also introduced me to Yogananda's spiritual community, the Self Realization Fellowship, and to the Self Realization Lake Shrine, in Malibu, not far from where I lived. The *Autobiography of a Yogi* answered so many of the questions, which I had had for years about Jesus, God, religion and the purpose of life. Yogananda's teachings included a distinction between Jesus, the person, and the state of "Christ consciousness," which He attained. He demonstrated through the examples of saints in his *Autobiography* and in his own life, that the state of "Christ consciousness" was something that all sincere Christians could not only aspire to, but realize within themselves through the practice of Kriya Yoga. This is what I had been searching for even as a young boy. I began attending church services at the SRF church in Malibu, studying lessons from the SRF Church's correspondence course, and meditating regularly. At the end of the summer, when I returned to Georgetown University, I began to seriously question my Christian faith. Who was Jesus? One of the most influential human beings of all times? The founder of Christianity? A messiah or savior sent by God to redeem humanity of its sins? What were His teachings? Is our knowledge of Jesus limited to what is recorded in the Bible? What has modern historical research to say about what Jesus did and taught?

I read many of the works of the "Fathers" of the early Christian Church in an attempt to answer the questions I had about "What did Jesus teach? What did He really say?" "What were the original teachings of Jesus, before the Christian religion became organized?" I came to the conclusion that in order to determine this I would have to learn Greek and perhaps ancient Aramaic, and become a scholar of the ancient texts that had recently been discovered in the Sinai Desert, like the Gospel of Thomas. Or, I reasoned, I could try to live my life the way Jesus did, with emphasis on the spiritual practices of the early Church Fathers, and so discover the original teachings of Jesus. I was being drawn into the spiritual experiences, which my deepening practice of meditation was providing to me, and so, I chose to enter the path of Classical Yoga. For the next thirty seven years I practiced Kriya Yoga, the form of Yoga that Yogananda pioneered in the West.

When I returned to Georgetown University in the fall of 1968, for my senior year, I experienced a personal crisis in faith. Who was Jesus? Who was Yogananda? What should I place my faith in? Was I still sure that I had made a good decision in taking up the practice of Yogananda's Kriya Yoga? I went to see Father King. I knew that he had read the *Autobiography of a Yogi*, and I knew I could trust his opinion about my dilemma. Then I asked him whether Yogananda, his teachings, and the path of Kriya Yoga, which I had recently dedicated myself to, were from God?

Father King reassured me that "Yogananda and his teachings were definitely from God," and that I could continue with them in full faith. "Follow your heart," he told me. He said that there was nothing to worry about and that I would be guided.

From this experience I learned that only wisdom was worth seeking. I renewed my resolve to "follow my heart," and plunged into the practice and teachings of Yogananda and Kriya Yoga.

My Initiation

At the end of 1969, I had passed the U.S. Foreign Service written and oral examinations, yet remained undecided about my future plans. One day I noticed an advertisement for a "Kriya Yoga" class in the local *Free Press,* and out of interest in Yogananda's teachings on Kriya Yoga attended it. Walking into the small apartment off Dupont Circle, I saw someone the likes of which I had never before seen. There, sitting on a low bench, was a small dark skinned man with a long beard and long hair, dressed only in a white cloth, from the waist down. But, more than his unique distinguishing features, I was amazed to see a tremendous glow of light around his body. It was like a cloud. He was sitting there quietly, waiting. There were two young men and two young women, his disciples sitting quietly on the floor in front of him. That evening he taught me a set of eighteen Yoga postures and gave an inspired lecture on "Babaji's Kriya Yoga," a "scientific art of God-Truth realization." His name was Yogi S.A.A. Ramaiah. Little did I know that this first meeting was to be the first of many over the next eighteen years. After attending every one of his monthly classes until the following May, I decided to receive initiation from him into the secret techniques of Kriya Yoga in June 1970, at his ashram in New York City. This decision was made after much reflection, as I had, the previous summer, submitted my application to enter the monastery of Yogananda's Self Realization Fellowship, in southern California. But, I did so, not only because I was drawn to this yogi as a "living" spiritual teacher, but also to the disciplined, yogic way of life "in the world," which his urban ashrams offered. The "initiation" into Kriya Yoga spanned several days of instruction and practice of a powerful breathing technique known as Kriya Kundalini Pranayama, and a series of progressive meditation techniques. The experience was wonderful, deeply moving and transforming. I felt as if I had finally found my path to God. The breathing technique enabled me to glimpse an inner light and a mental stillness. In this stillness, Yogi Ramaiah's often quoted dictum from the Psalms, "Be Still and Know that I am God," assumed real significance. My future plans of Foreign Service began to take shape in an entirely new direction.

Shortly, after graduation from Georgetown University, I felt the resolve to settle fulltime into living a spiritual life and to join a Kriya Yoga ashram in southern California. Before allowing me to do so, however, Yogiar, as we fondly called him asked me to attempt a three month probationary period during which I was required to practice the Kriya Yoga techniques I had learned for eight hours per day, work for eight hours per day, and use the remaining eight hours per day for daily routine activities and rest. In addition, I was asked to observe one day of silence and fasting every week, eat only vegetarian food, and live a simple, yogic way of life. If I could do this on my own, I would be allowed to continue this disciplined way of life in one of his ashrams. Over the next three months, practicing the techniques I had learned, I gradually increased my capacity to fulfill these requirements, in a rented room in a house across from Georgetown University's Hospital, and while working in the nearby Saville Bookstore. After three months, I drove across country and was permitted to join his ashram, two small apartments, in Downey, California, which I shared with him and several other disciples.

This yogic discipline and way of life was designed to purify my consciousness of its past associations and tendencies, and secondly to enable me to make a contribution to society from the perspective of a new spiritual consciousness. Like the Gnostics, who believed that one could know God inwardly, through secret, powerful spiritual practices taught in initiations, I felt myself coming closer to a realization of the Divine. During altered states of consciousness brought about through the practices of Kriya Yoga, I realized myself as a vast luminous being of light, formless and timeless, bliss itself. However, regardless of how deep my mind would drop into these states, my mind and body would repeatedly bring me back into the ordinary state of consciousness, filled with worldly preoccupations. How was I to overcome this difficulty, going back and forth, in and out of these exalted states of bliss?

During this first year, Yogiar inspired me to study the writings of the Siddha Thirumular, and the works of Sri Aurobindo, the Indian sage who spoke of the "supramental" transformation of humanity. But unlike the Gnostics, who rejected the world, as inherently evil, Yogi Ramaiah, Sri Aurobindo and the Yoga Siddhas taught that the world was implicitly Divine, and that it was the world, which could and should be transformed, beginning with our self. And it was viewed from this new perspective, that the teachings of Jesus assumed a new meaning for me. It was purification of my human nature that became the key. I rejected the old dualistic choice between the spiritual and the material, and began to embrace both. My spiritual practices had revealed to me that God was no longer only "out there," but also "here within." My dilemmas and choices paralleled in many ways what many early Christians must have had, as they tried to reconcile competing interpretations of the teachings of Jesus, and various paths to salvation proclaimed by early forms of Christianity.

In 1971, I was initiated into a powerful series of advanced techniques, after I had fulfilled many strenuous preconditions. I had to practice the techniques I had learned in the first and second initiations for at least fifty-six hours per week, for a total of fifty-two weeks, among other things, all the while fulfilling my obligations to work full time and perform community service. During that year, I worked as a social worker first, in Long Beach, California and then in Chicago, where I was sent to open a new Kriya Yoga Center. I was then asked to save five thousand dollars in order to go to India for a year, where I was to engage in intensive Yoga practice.

Arriving in India, I quickly settled into a routine of yogic practice in the ashram, which had been established near Yogi Ramaiah's ancestral home, in the Chettinad area of Tamil Nadu. Alone, visited only by a servant who prepared my meals and cleaned, with no distractions (and no plumbing, and very little electricity) my aspirations to know God roared and soared. My call met with a response: a series of powerful meditation experiences, which filled me great peace and joy. Although nearly impossible to describe, because they did not involve "forms" or "visions," but the expansion of my consciousness itself, I can recall how immediate was the Presence of the Lord and even amidst the most mundane activities of daily life: while bathing, as water poured over me at the well, eating the simple, spicy vegetarian curry and rice cooked over a dung fire, bumping along in a country bus to the nearby town of Karaikudi, bowing as I passed local temples, and reflected in the bright eyes of the local children who came to the ashram for Yoga classes and even in the sugar candy they were given to savor afterwards. I felt that I had entered, at times, a timeless realm, so great was the peace. The events in themselves were nothing out of the ordinary, but were beheld with the perspective of ever-renewing joy. God was everywhere in that simple life with the ever-present bliss.

Returning to America was a bit of a culture shock. However, from 1972 to 1995 I worked as an economist, and in fact my first job was for the Department of Defense, in the Pentagon. In 1977, I immigrated to Canada, and worked in industry in Montreal. During all of these years I lived in the Yoga ashrams practicing Kriya Yoga an average of eight hours per day. During this period I also traveled again to India and to Sri Lanka for two year long retreats, in 1980 to 1981 and from 1986 to 1987 where I engaged in non-stop intensive yogic practice.

Spiritual energy ripens as fruit ripens, and at the proper moment, the fruit and the seed drop from the tree that gave it nourishment and find new fertile soil, which enable it to grow. On Christmas Eve, 1988, in a series of profound spiritual experiences, it became clear that I was to leave my teacher's ashram and organization and begin to initiate others into Kriya Yoga. The message was unmistakable, and impossible to ignore. I had never dreamed of leaving the community, which had nurtured me for the previous eighteen years. Until then, no student had been authorized to teach anything more than the eighteen postures of Kriya Hatha Yoga. To take responsibility for initiating others was a huge responsibility. However, on January 2, 1984, after Yogi Ramaiah suffered a heart attack, he gave me a stringent set of conditions to fulfill, and told me that if I succeeded, I would be authorized to initiate others into the 144 Kriyas, or techniques of Kriya Yoga. This request had come as a surprise. I could only assume that it was because I had honored all of the conditions asked of me, and practiced the techniques of Kriya Yoga for at least fifty-six hours per week without a break for more than twelve years, an ideal period of which Yogiar had often spoken. It took me another three years to fulfill all of the additional conditions. When I had done so, I informed Yogi Ramaiah, and he instructed me simply to wait. Two years later, the message came. Yogiar had often said that once he had brought us to the feet of the "Guru," his work with us would be completed.

Henceforward, my life was directed by the Light of the Guru,(a persistant inspiration and intuition, filled with insight). It was also focused on "showing the path to others." Beginning in 1989, my life moved in this new direction; doors opened, and everything facilitated my new mission. I began to share Kriya Yoga with others, first, on weekends, in Montreal, after later, after the publication of my first book on Kriya Yoga, to persons all over the world. Ever since it has been a joy for me to share this "light," this precious spiritual science, with more than 10,000 students in more than twenty countries, and to train over a dozen teachers to do the same.

A few years ago, I read a cover story in *Time Magazine* about how scholars had determined which words attributed to Jesus in the Bible, were considered to be authentic, based upon critical scientific methods and examination of ancient manuscripts. The Time article spoke of three levels of authenticity regarding the words attributed to Jesus. I had myself been engaged in research to preserve, transcribe, translate, authenticate, comment upon and publish the ancient manuscripts of the Yoga Siddhas - ancient adepts and contemporaries of, and not unlike, Jesus. I founded and sponsored the Yoga Siddha Research Centre in Chennai, whose director, Dr. T.N. Ganapathy, along with a team of six scholars has published six volumes of the Siddhas' works since 2000. Then, two years ago, I decided to return to my original quest: the teachings of Jesus. What had the scholars found about what Jesus really said? I had no preconceptions. I knew that there would undoubtedly be surprises. My training and experience as a social scientist helped me to frame my questions as hypotheses and to accept as true only those answers that could be supported by the data. When I found what scholars in the Jesus Seminar, Elaine Pagels and Bart Ehrman had written, I felt that I had perhaps found some missing pieces to a puzzle, which had eluded me as a young man at Georgetown. More importantly, from my perspective, I saw direct comparisons between the wisdom teachings of Jesus and those of the Yoga Siddhas, hundreds of years prior to the birth of Jesus, as well as ever since. To share and reaffirm this timeless wisdom in a modern context is my purpose in writing this book. What follows is the result of my comparison of these teachings in a very personal and renewed search as a Christian.

INTRODUCTION

Questions

Who was Jesus? One of the most influential human beings of all times? The founder of Christianity? A *messiah* or savior sent by God to redeem humanity of its sins? What were His teachings? Is our knowledge of Jesus limited to what is recorded in the Bible? What has modern historical research to say about what Jesus did and taught? Have there been other spiritual masters in India whose teachings are similar to those of Jesus? If so, what light can they shed on the teachings of Jesus?

With the discovery of many new source documents in the Sinai Desert and near the Dead Sea, and with the advent of modern methods of textual analysis by scholars who are independent of institutional bias, today most Biblical scholars will agree that the books of the Bible's New Testament are written at several levels of authenticity:

- What were likely the actual words of Jesus, quoted in the gospels of Matthew, Mark and Luke, but recorded several decades afterwards.
- What were likely interpolations - words attributed to Jesus by unknown sources.
- What was said about Jesus or about his teachings by others, for example, Paul in his "letters," which make up most of the rest of the New Testament, and which served as the basis for early Church dogma.

Within Christianity and in the popular understanding of Jesus and his teaching, how much have these interpolations and early Church dogma distorted or obscured the actual words and teachings of Jesus? What do the actual words of Jesus say about who Jesus was and what his teachings were? What do the actual words of Jesus not say? Answers to these questions are a prerequisite to making comparisons between the teachings of Jesus and the teachings of the Gnostics and other mystics, such as those of the Yoga Siddhas. Previous attempts by some, including Swami Prabhavananda's *The Sermon on the Mount According to Vedanta*, and Paramahansa Yogananda's *The Second Coming of Christ* made comparisons with Christianity's dogma reflected in the King James version of the Bible. They did not consider the work of biblical historians who have suggested numerous inaccuracies in this English version of the Bible, in comparison with the original Greek. They do not take into consideration the many findings that modern critical historical research has brought to light. Yogananda interpreted who Jesus was, by distinguishing "Jesus" the person from "Christ" the state of "consciousness," which he had attained. Most of his interpretation was based upon statements allegedly made by Jesus, for example, the "I am" statements, in the Gospel of John, which most critical scholars now consider to be interpolations and words not spoken by Jesus. This present work presents a comparison between the teachings of the Yoga Siddhas, with those of the teachings that are considered now to be the most authentic teachings of Jesus, based upon the results of modern, critical, historical research.

Others have attempted to compare what Jesus did with what other saints, prophets and sages have done. Some have speculated that Jesus went to India or Tibet, where he was initiated into their sacred traditions. Holger Kersten, for example, in his *Jesus Lived in India,* assembled many arguments, based upon very little evidence that Jesus not only went to India prior to his crucifixion, but returned there and died in Kashmir. He concluded however, that we really do not know what Jesus did.

As we will see, modern historical scholars have been able to form a broad consensus about what Jesus taught, but history provides little evidence of what Jesus actually did. Nothing is recorded about the so called "missing years" of Jesus between the recorded incidents in the temple in Jerusalem, when, at the age of twelve, he spoke authoritatively to the scribes and Pharisees, and his appearance at the age of 30, when he begins his mission, by the Sea of Galilee. Therefore, we must look elsewhere to understand the influences that transformed Jesus, the carpenter's son from Nazareth, into the Messiah, or savior of the Jewish people, and the Christ, revered by millions ever since.

But there are other sources, which by comparison with what Jesus said and taught and how he lived, clearly indicate what those influences were. Examples include the writings of the Gnostics, discovered at Nag Hammadi, in the Sinai, in 1945, the Jewish Essenes, discovered at Qumram in 1948 and thousands of ancient documents which trace the development of early Christianity, and which portray its competing divisions.

Several scholars have studied the Yoga Siddhas of India: Eliade, Briggs, Zvelebil, Ganapathy, White, Govindan, Feuerstein, in particular. A critical edition of the most important work of the Tamil Yoga Siddhas, the *Tirumandiram*, by the Siddha Tirumular (written between the 2nd century B.C. and the fourth century C.E.) was produced by the Tamil scholar Suba Annamalai in 2000, from thirteen existing manuscripts. A new English language translation and commentary of this critical edition of the *Tirumandiram* is currently being prepared by a team of scholars lead by Dr. T.N. Ganapathy. Most recently, the research of the Yoga Siddha Research Centre in Chennai, India, lead by Dr. T.N. Ganapathy, has brought out a series of books providing, for the first time, translation and commentary of the Yoga Siddhas, or "perfected" yogis of South India, who were contemporaries of Jesus. Their teachings and miraculous powers were remarkably similar to those of Jesus. This makes possible an intriguing comparison between the teachings and miracles of Jesus and those of the Yoga Siddhas.

The writings of the South India Yoga Siddhas have been largely ignored until recently. They were not well preserved by the orthodox institutions because of the Siddhas' severe condemnation of the caste system, excessive emphasis on temple worship and scriptures, and the authority of the Brahmins, the priestly caste, which monopolized religious affairs in India. The writings of the Siddhas were in the vernacular language of the people rather than Sanskrit. Knowledge of Sanskrit was limited for the most part to the Brahmin caste, whose priests and scholars dominated the religious and educational systems. The Siddhas condemned this monopoly of the Brahmins, and taught that the Lord could only be known by *Jnana Yoga*, wisdom born of self-knowledge, meditation and other spiritual practices, particularly through *Kundalini Yoga*. Many in the orthodox caste, the Brahmins, reacted by burning the writings of the Siddhas and sought to prejudice popular opinion against the Siddhas by ridiculing them. The writings of the Siddhas were written in what is referred to as a "twilight language," which deliberately obscures its deeper meaning to all but Yoga initiates. This great gap in scholarly understanding of the Siddhas writings, however, has recently begun to be filled by a series of books, produced by a team of leading scholars working for the Yoga Siddha Research Centre in Chennai, India. The Centre has collected, preserved, transcribed and begun to translate thousands of palm leaf manuscripts written by the Yoga Siddhas, which had been all but forgotten in several manuscript libraries of southern India.

Remarkable Similarities

Even a cursory comparison of the teachings of Jesus and those of the *Siddhas* by anyone familiar with the two reveals remarkable similarities:

- Jesus taught in parables, metaphor, paradox, and parody, conveying profound teachings in a way that illiterate listeners could easily understand and remember. He was an iconoclast, who sought to move His listeners to realize the spirit, not merely the letter of the Jewish law and worship practices.

- The Yoga Siddhas taught in the form of poems, in the vernacular language of the illiterate people, in a way that they could easily understand, memorize and recall. Several layers of meaning could be attributed to both the teachings of Jesus and the Siddhas. The deepest layers could be understood only by the initiate, who had been taught by a spiritual master how to access the inner reality through such practices as meditation and silence.

- Jesus severely condemned the Pharisees and the merchants in the temple, physically assaulting their shops. When challenged by the Pharisees on what authority did he speak, he replied: "I shall destroy this temple, and within three days, raise it up!" His resurrection from the cross proved His point, that the real temple is within oneself.

The Yoga Siddhas also condemned emphasis on temple worship and idol worship. Nowhere in any of their writings do they sing in praise of any of the popular *Hindu* deities or images of God. They taught that the human body is the true temple of God and it is only through a process of inner purification that one can come to know the Lord.

- Neither Jesus nor the Siddhas intended to create a new religion. They taught that God is present in the world. They taught how to realize God through self discipline and self awareness, and through our connection to others.

- Jesus taught forgiveness of sins or transgressions. One of his most important parables, that of the prodigal son, exemplifies this.

The Siddhas taught how to "detach" from the influence of *samskaras* (subconscious tendencies), which collectively are referred to as karma (the consequences of actions, words and thoughts). Forgiveness and dispassion are synonymous at a deep level of understanding, and central to both the teachings of Jesus and such Siddhas as Patanjali.

- Jesus repeatedly referred to himself modestly as the "son of man," but later, the writers of the Gospels, as well as Paul referred to him as "son of God."

The Siddhas distinguished, the "lower self," the body-mind-personality, held together by egoism (*asmita*), from the higher

- In what scholars consider to be the most authentic parts of the New Testament, the three synoptic Gospels, Mark, Matthew and Luke, Jesus says little about himself and when He does, it is always modestly.

The Siddhas also have little to say about themselves in their writings. They spoke of freeing themselves from ignorance, egoism and delusion. Consequently, they enjoyed an expanded consciousness and became instruments of the Divine, working "miracles."

- Jesus taught that the Lord, whom he referred to as the Father, not only existed, but that He loves you. He also taught that to know Him, one must overcome egoism and attachment to the things of this world.

The Siddhas also taught that by a progressive process of self study, discipline and purification, one can realize the Lord. They did not fear the Lord. They loved Him. To them, God was Love and Love was God. Surrender to the Lord was the means of their progressive transformation. They realized the Lord as Absolute Being, Consciousness and Bliss within themselves.

- Jesus repeatedly emphasized that "the Kingdom of Heaven is within you." The theme of Jesus' teachings in the synoptic gospels as well as the Gospel of St Thomas is "the Kingdom of Heaven." But in the Epistles of Paul, as well as the Gospel of John, which are considered by the vast majority of reputable scholars to contain only interpolations (statements put into the mouth of Jesus by unknown sources) the theme is Jesus himself, his mission and his person.

The Siddhas repeatedly taught that the Lord was to be found within oneself, as Absolute Being, Consciousness and Bliss, and that this state could only be realized through the cultivation of *samadhi* (God consciousness). This is not a creation of the mind. It is the realization of the Divine Witness within, and the cultivation of a divine life, from the perspective of this God consciousness. They taught that the Lord is, unlike our soul, unaffected by desires and *karma*. Being one with everything, the Siddhas retained no more inclination to be of special personage. The Siddhas rarely spoke of their person, and they never encouraged the worship of their person, but rather of that omnipresent Reality within them.

- Jesus used the metaphor of Light to represent consciousness of his true identity; "when thine eye is single, thy whole body shall be full of light." (Luke 11.34)

The Siddhas referred to the Supreme Being as all pervasive light or as the supreme grace light. They referred to the Supreme Being as *Shiva Shakti* (Conscious Energy), and taught that it could be realized within oneself as the sublime, divine *kundalini* light energy within the subtle body.

- Jesus was reported to have ascended bodily into heaven 40 days after he rose from the dead. During these 40 days he appeared to his disciples. Doubting Thomas verified his corporeal nature by touching his hands. The body of Jesus was not buried.

The Siddhas sing repeatedly of their total surrender to the Lord, a surrender, which includes the very cells of their physical body, which creates a transformation begetting immortality.

- Jesus was reportedly opposed and crucified by those who ruled the temple founded by David in Jerusalem - the priests and Pharisees. They saw him as a threat to their privileged position. Jesus sought to liberate the Jews not from the Romans, but from their spiritual ignorance, fear, and domination by the priests. He taught them through his parables, and initiated chosen disciples into how to know God by turning within, in esoteric practices.

The Siddhas have been opposed to this day by the vested interests of Hinduism, the Brahmins, who control the temples and serve as intermediaries between the common person and the "gods" of the Hindu pantheon. The Siddhas are condemned and ridiculed as "miracle workers," fakirs and worse, by the Brahmins, who fear their popular appeal among the masses. The Siddhas and other yogic adepts initiate the most qualified students into the esoteric practices of Kundalini Yoga and meditation.

- Jesus emphasized love and the inner experience or communion with God, rather than the law of the Old Testament.

The Siddhas rejected the Vedic scripture's emphasis on external fire sacrifice and ritual; they emphasized the inner path to the Lord through love and *Yoga*.

- Jesus performed many miracles as a result of his powers, or *siddhis*.

So did the Siddhas. The ordinary person dissipates their energy through the senses, attracted by desires. When one realizes the Presence of the Lord within, one gains access to unlimited power and consciousness. Unmanifest and potential, it is known as *kundalini*. When it is awakened, one becomes an instrument of the Divine.

- Jesus spent 40 days in the wilderness in meditation and prayer, and as a result acquired great powers.

The Siddhas performed similar *tapas* (penance) with resulting *siddhis* (powers). Even the number 40 is of particular significance with regard to a period of practice of penance in the yogic tradition.

- Both the Siddhas and Jesus exhibited great social concern. Jesus left John the Baptist, and returned to the urban areas and consorted with tax collectors and other disreputable types. He encouraged counter-cultural movements against established tradition.

The Siddhas sought to show the path to the Lord to everyone, by teaching what one must do, especially through Yoga and hygienic living standards and medicine, and also what one must avoid.

- Jesus accepted Mary Magdalene as a disciple when he allowed her to wash and to anoint his feet. He initiated his most worthy disciples, like Thomas, into esoteric teachings, which enabled them to realize the Supreme Being, beyond the creator God.

The Siddhas showed their surrender to their Gurus by washing, anointing or touching their feet. They initiated their disciples into advanced techniques of Yoga to expand their consciousness and bring about Self realization.

- Jesus was not merely a teacher or rabbi to his disciples, but a God-man, who remained an enigma to all of his direct disciples. They struggled to comprehend his teachings, his parables, and referred to him variously as a prophet or the Messiah, the anointed one who would deliver them from the yoke of Roman tyranny. Their confusion lead to the formation of a multiplicity of sects in early Christianity, until the fourth century C.E., when the Church, in alliance with the Roman emperor, seeking to unify Christianity and the Roman Empire, defined Christian dogma and creeds, and declared as heretics those who did not adhere to its dogma.

The Siddhas were Gurus (dispellers of darkness) who showed the path to the Lord, and were also revered as ones who embodied divinity. They extolled the authority of one's own inner spiritual experience, rather than the authority of the *Vedas* (scriptures). For this reason, the orthodox condemned them. The Siddhas continue to be an enigma for most Hindus.

In this work we will explore and compare these and other areas, which will shed great light on the questions "Who was Jesus?" And "How can I best understand His teachings?"

Why Should Christians Study Yoga?

The short answer is that the study and practice of Yoga will make a Christian a better Christian. Also, because it will provide valuable spiritual experience, mental peace, energy and good health, all essential in realizing the goals of both persons of faith and rationalists. Just as the Buddha was not a Buddhist, Jesus was not a Christian. The Buddha was certainly a yogi, who undertook to find the cause of human suffering, and the remedy for it, through philosophical enquiry. Who am I? Where have I come from and where am I going? Why is there evil? What is there after this life? In that way Yoga can be considered to be the practical side of all religions. It contains no dogma, no limiting beliefs. It is not a religion. It may be considered to be an "open philosophy" for it accepts various approaches to Truth.

It is widely recognized to be one of the six main systems of philosophy in India. As such it fits perfectly into Pope John Paul II's recommendation that Christians study philosophy, including the Eastern philosophies, in order to become better Christians. His Papal Encyclical "Faith and Reason" provides the long answer to the above question. In it Pope John Paul II argues that:

"In both East and West, we may trace a journey which has led humanity down the centuries to meet and engage truth more and more deeply. It is a journey which has unfolded—as it must—within the horizon of personal self-consciousness: the more human beings know reality and the world, the more they know themselves in their uniqueness, with the question of the meaning of things and of their very existence becoming ever more pressing. This is why all that is the object of our knowledge becomes a part of our life. The admonition "Know yourself" was carved on the temple portal at Delphi, as testimony to a basic truth to be adopted as a minimal norm by those who seek to set themselves apart from the rest of creation as "human beings," that is, as those who "know themselves.""[1]

Yoga is a means to "know thyself." From the grossest to the most subtle levels, Yoga gives us the means to reach the highest and most ethereal subtleties of material substance. Yoga can take us beyond the grasp of our senses, the thoughts of our mind, and even beyond our most subtle consciousness to the Force-Love beyond it. Yoga examines the fundamental principles and laws of the cosmos, their purpose and their demand on divine evolution. It examines how the principle of grace works in life through the physical instrument, through the mind, the physical nervous system and vital organs.

Yoga can teach us how to embrace the suffering of our life and to overcome it. The Siddhas were neither pessimistic nor illusionist. They saw the world as a mixture of division, darkness, limitation, desire, struggle, pain and splendor, beauty and truth. They recognized the mind as an instrument of the soul imprisoned in it. The view "I am" is a force of creative power possessed by the soul to lift it from this prison. The profound realization of "I am" is a powerful means to knowing ourselves truly as children of God. According to the Siddhas, we share consciousness with God. But rare is the person who understands and imbibes this Truth. God is behind all that exists as the Eternal Witness. But that Supreme Consciousness can perfectly express itself in this manifest world only in one who has integrally harmonized Truth within itself. A Siddha is one who has done so, drawing body and soul into a new identification with absolute perfection. This occurs only after having discarded all identification with the mind's imperfect state of physical manifestation and consciousness. A Siddha has surrendered to the Supreme Consciousness at all levels, from the spiritual to the physical. Jesus could be identified as one such a being. He stepped out of the imperfect human form to enter a new Consciousness and Being.

Yoga teaches that the imperfect reality of human existence is seen only by the mind, the limited mind of desire, division, darkness, struggle, and pain. And to overcome it, the mind itself must reach a psychic aspiration towards perfection lying beyond itself. The mind of a man must seek union with an Ideal of perfection and harmonize itself totally with it. This process requires complete surrender to the Supreme Being, Consciousness and Bliss.

The Objectives of This Book

This book is addressed to the following readers:

1. Christians who are interested in comparing Eastern spiritual teachings with those of Christianity.
2. Students of spiritual Yoga, otherwise known as Classical Yoga and Tantra, as well students and practitioners of meditation and other spiritual disciplines.
3. Serious Biblical students, including those interested in the question "What did Jesus really teach, before the formation of Christian dogma?"

The objectives of this book are to

1. Demonstrate that what Jesus taught, for example through his parables and sayings, was amazingly similar to what the Yoga masters, the Siddhas, taught.
2. To explore the implications of these parallel teachings for those seeking to apply them in their own life, not so much to know about God, as to how to know God through higher states of consciousness.
3. To show how the discoveries of ancient manuscripts, and their analysis by independent critical scholars using scientific methods, provide much insight into the original teachings of Jesus.
4. To demonstrate why the "sayings" of Jesus, circulated orally during the first decades following his crucifixion before being recorded, are probably the most authentic source of his teachings that we have available today. These are limited to a few dozen parables, aphorisms and sharp retorts, which were repeated in the oral tradition for two or three decades before they were eventually recorded by the anonymous writers of the Gospels.

5. To show how the original teachings of Jesus, as recorded in his "sayings" and parables, became obscured once Christianity was defined in terms of dogmas and creeds.
6. To explore the question "Who was Jesus?" based upon those statements that many modern critical scholars have concluded are the most authentic.
7. To explore the questions "Where is the Kingdom of God?" and "How may I reach it?" based upon those statements that many modern critical scholars have concluded are the most authentic.
8. To explore the question "Why are the teachings of Jesus so contrary to ordinary human nature?"

CHAPTER 1

Modern Historical Research of Jesus and Early Christianity

The modern historical quest of Jesus began in the Renaissance with Galileo, Copernicus, Kepler and Newton and the dawn of reason, research and science. Until then, Church dogma and creed was considered fact. The Church taught that the world was flat. Galileo with his telescope proved that it was round. A increasing desire to put all knowledge to the test led to the development of modern historical research. The scientific method began separating the factual from the fictional in accounts of the past.

In the 1700's Herman Reimarus (1694-1768), a professor of oriental languages in Hamburg, Germany, made the first effort to distinguish what Jesus himself said and what was said in the Christian creeds. However, it was Thomas Jefferson, the author of the American Declaration of Independence, one of the "founding fathers of the United States of America" and its third President, who made one of the first serious efforts to determine what he called the authentic accounts and sayings of Jesus. Jefferson began this work late in the first of his two terms as President, and finished it more than 12 years later, in 1816. He cut out those passages, which he considered authentic from the King James Version of the Bible, and pasted them in chronological order on blank sheets, along with the Greek translation, later adding the French and Latin translations. The result, "The Life and Morals of Jesus of Nazareth" remained with his family until 1904, when it was published by order of the Congress of the United States, and a copy was given to all members of the House and Senate.

In private correspondence with his former political rival, ex-president John Adams, he wrote:

"To the corruption of Christianity I am, indeed, opposed; but not to the genuine precepts of Jesus himself. I am a Christian in the only sense in which he wanted anyone to be: sincerely attached to his doctrines, in preference to all others; ascribing to himself every *human* excellence; and believing he never claimed any other… The whole history of these books (the Gospels) is so defective and doubtful that it seems vain to attempt minute enquiry into it: and such tricks have been played with their text, and with the texts of other books relating to them, that we have a right, from that cause, to entertain much doubt what parts of them are genuine. In the New Testament there is internal evidence that parts of it have proceeded from an extraordinary man; and that other parts are of the fabric of very inferior minds. It is as easy to separate those parts, as to pick out diamonds from dunghills."[1]

In another letter to John Adams dated October 12, 1813, he wrote:

"We must reduce our volume to the simple Evangelist; select even from them, the very words only of Jesus, paring off the amphibologisms into which they have been led by forgetting often, or not understanding, what had fallen from him, by giving their own misconceptions as his dicta, and expressing unintelligibly for others what they had not understood themselves. There will be found remaining the most sublime and benevolent code of morals which has ever been offered to man."[2]

Jefferson was shocked and offended that the words of Jesus had been altered so much. All reputable scholars today, however, recognize that the official Gospels were compiled in Greek, many decades after the death of Jesus, by persons who had never heard them in their original

Aramaic. Furthermore, all reputable scholars today agree that much of what Jesus was supposed to have said really originated in the very different teachings of the early Church. What was originally the Gospel, or "good news," the wisdom teachings of Jesus was largely replaced or obscured by teachings *about* Jesus even in the most authentic parts of the New Testament: Mark, Matthew and Luke.

The Development of the Seven Pillars of Modern Historical Biblical Research

Many critical scholars of biblical history have come to a consensus in their findings about the teachings of Jesus and the origins of the New Testament. Before discussing in the next section, how this consensus came about, and the methods of modern critical historical research, I would like to summarize their findings. These are summarized below, and are known as the "Seven Pillars of Modern Historical Biblical Research: "

1. The views of Reimarus, mentioned above, and his successors, lead David Friedrich Strauss to write "Life of Jesus Critically Examined" in 1835. In its 1,400 pages, Strauss made a clear distinction between the historical Jesus and what he termed the "mythical" one. He defined the latter as anything legendary or supernatural. In other words, a distinction was made between the Christ of faith as encapsulated in the early creeds, and the historical Jesus, as revealed by modern methods of research and excavation.

2. The recognition that the three Gospels, namely, Matthew, Mark and Luke were much closer to the historical Jesus than was the fourth Gospel, John, which presented a "spiritual" Jesus. These three Synoptic Gospels (Greek *synoptikós* – "equivalent to" or "seen together") are so named because of their close similarities which permits the texts to be set out in parallel for comparison. They provide parallel accounts of the life of Jesus.

3. Further research led to the recognition that the Gospel of Mark is older than that of Matthew or Luke.

4. The recognition of a hypothetical source, referred to as "Q" to explain why Matthew and Luke have material in common beyond their dependence upon Mark, lead to the so called "double tradition:" that Matthew and Luke were based upon Mark and Q.

5. The recognition that Jesus had rejected the teachings, promoted by John the Baptist, that the end of the world was at hand. Modern historical research was originally dominated by the rise of a view of the "eschatological Jesus," by Albert Schweitzer in his "The Quest of the Historical Jesus" (1906) and Johannes Weiss in his "Jesus' Proclamation of the Kingdom of God" (1892). They believed that Jesus had proclaimed that the age was going to come to an end in a cataclysmic event, known as the *eschaton* (Greek – "last event"). The "eschatological Jesus" reigned supreme among Gospel scholars until the end of World War II. Conservative and neo-orthodox views, as expressed by Karl Barth and Rudolf Bultmann also stifled any real interest in the historical Jesus from 1920 to 1970. They dismissed the quest for the historical Jesus as an "illegitimate" attempt to develop a factual basis for faith – "an attempt to prove Christian claims made on behalf of Jesus." To this day, historical studies of Christian origins must labor under this theological condemnation.

Since the 1970's, modern biblical research shifted away from its earlier academic nests in the church, seminaries and isolated theological settings. It became free of neo-orthodox and eschatological views. The fifth pillar was established: it was John the Baptist who had proclaimed the end of the world, and Jesus' disciples had acquired this view from the Baptist movement. Jesus himself appears to have rejected apocalyptic prophesy. He does not refer to it in his parables. His vision of God's domain was that it was modest and yet pervasive. What need had God for an apocalyptic event? He returned from the desert to urban centers to associate with even the most socially unacceptable persons - tax collectors, prostitutes, and sinners developing a message, not of the end of the world, but of the presence of the Kingdom of Heaven within and all around us. But his ministry lasted less than two years, and many of his disciples had formerly been disciples of John the Baptist. After Jesus' departure, his disciples reverted to the teachings of John the Baptist, and overlaid upon them the tradition of sayings and parables and "memories" of Jesus. They bolstered this with references to the Jewish prophecies, and the Jew's longing for one who would overthrow the Romans' domination of ancient Israel. The disciples thus made Jesus a cult figure similar to others in Greek mystery religions, and constructed out of their own growing conviction of Jesus, that he was the *messiah* (Hebrew - *māshīaḥ* "anointed [one]"), come to save them. The quest for the historical Jesus is therefore an attempt to distinguish a forgotten Jesus from the literary figure portrayed in the Gospels.

6. The distinction between the oral culture in which Jesus taught with short, provocative, memorable, often-repeated phrases and stories, versus the print culture, which continues to this day.

7. The final pillar is the reversal of the earlier burden of proof. It is now assumed that the Gospels are "narratives in which the memory of Jesus is embellished by mythic elements that express the church's faith in him, and by plausible fictions that enhance the telling of the Gospel story for first century listeners who knew about divine men and miracle workers first hand."[3] Historical elements in the narratives must be demonstrated to be so. This reverses the earlier Orthodox view that the Gospels were 100% historically accurate, but also allows for the investigation of data preserved in the Gospels that may be historically accurate.

These seven pillars cannot guarantee a historically accurate view of Jesus. But neither can those of the numerous sects within Christianity. The latter's view of Jesus varies with the theological perspective of the advocates of each sect.

Methodology and Findings of Modern Critical Biblical Scholars

The consensus among most critical biblical historians, discussed above, was expressed in a significant study known as the Jesus Seminar, wherein over two hundred biblical historians, including some of the most prominent scholars, voted on the degree of authenticity for every phrase in the four canonical Gospels and the Gospel of Thomas. They inventoried, classified and then critically examined all the words attributed to Jesus during the first three centuries of the Common Era - up to the year 313 C.E., when Emperor Constantine issued the Edict of Toleration. After the Council of Nicaea in 325 C.E. the Christianity was solidified in an Orthodox form, and other wings of the Christian movement that refused to conform, were gradually destroyed. The inventory of more than 1,500 items covers all the surviving Gospels and historical reports from the period. The goal of the seminar was to review each of the 1,500 items and determine which of them could be ascribed with a high degree of probability to Jesus, based upon rules of written and oral evidence. The items passing the test would be included in a database for determining who Jesus was and what he said. But the interpretation of the data was to be excluded from the agenda, and left to the individual scholars working from their own perspectives.

Voting was adopted, after extended debate, as the most efficient way of ascertaining whether a scholarly consensus existed on a given point. Voting, while it does not determine the truth, does indicate what the best judgment is of a significant number of scholars. The second agreement made by the scholars was to create a critical red letter edition of the Gospels as the vehicle of its public report. Fellows were permitted to cast ballots in secret under two different options for understanding the four colors:

Option 1:

>Red: I would include this item unequivocally in the database for determining who Jesus was.

>Pink: I would include this item with reservations (or modifications) in the database.

>Gray: I would not include this item in the database, but I might make use of some of the content in determining who Jesus was.

>Black: I would not include this item in the primary database.

Option 2:

>Red: Jesus undoubtedly said this or something very like it.

Pink: Jesus probably said something like this.

Gray: Jesus did not say this, but the ideas contained in it are close to His own.

Black: Jesus did not say this; it represents the perspective or content of a later or different tradition.

An unofficial interpretation of the colors was:

Red: That's Jesus.

Pink: Sure sounds like Jesus.

Gray: Well, maybe.

Black: There's been some mistake.

Rankings of verses was voted by weighted vote.

Red = 3

Pink = 2

Gray = 1

Black = 0

Before going into the results of this important study, it is important to understand the methodology by which scholars have come to their conclusions. In the chapter entitled "What Did Jesus Really Say?" the results will be discussed in detail. It is sufficient to mention at this point, however, that eighty two percent of the words ascribed to Jesus in the four canonical Gospels were not actually spoken by Him, according to the Jesus Seminar[4]. The more than two hundred Fellows of the Jesus Seminar are critical scholars, which means that they weighed empirical, factual evidence, open to confirmation by independent, neutral observers, which is the controlling factor in historical judgments. Non-critical scholars are those who put dogmatic considerations first and insist that the factual evidence confirm theological premises. Critical scholars adopt the principle of methodological skepticism: accept only what passes the rigorous tests of the rules of evidence. Critical scholars work from ancient texts in their original languages, in the case of the Gospels, in Greek, Coptic, Aramaic, Hebrew, Latin, and other tongues. Critical scholars practice their craft by submitting their work to the judgment of peers. Untested work is not highly regarded. The scholarship represented by the Fellows of the Jesus Seminar is the kind that has come to prevail in all the great universities of the world. Critical scholarship is regularly under attack by conservative Christian groups, who refuse to examine their own dogmas and belief systems in light of the findings of critical scholarship.

Among the criticisms made of the Jesus Seminar are accusations that it should not have excluded apocalyptic messages from the ministry of Jesus, that the findings largely represent the initial premises of the participants in the Seminar, that only about fourteen of the two hundred scholars are professors of biblical history in the most important universities, and that the fellows do not represent a fair cross-section of viewpoints. Members of the Jesus Seminar have responded to their critics in various books and dialogues, defending both their methodology and their conclusions.

In weighing these arguments, I have come to the conclusion that the criticisms are largely unwarranted, and that the consensus of participants in the Jesus Seminar is credible. The most serious criticism, that the findings largely represent the initial premises of the participants of the seminar, is defensible. Every investigation begins with a statement of hypotheses, rules of evidence and assumptions. The Jesus Seminar stated these explicitly, and applied its rules of evidence to the evidence available. Its rules of evidence were reasonable. Its basic premise was that unless a New Testament passage cannot be supported by the rules of evidence, it cannot be considered to have had the highest level of authenticity. Moreover, history, unlike science, is based upon the judgment of what probably happened, given the evidence available. The Jesus Seminar makes no claim to certainty. It expresses probability. Its' results represent the considered judgment of its participants. Furthermore, where there is no evidence, one cannot even make a judgment; therefore the Jesus Seminar was correct in limiting its examination to originality of the words in the New Testament, and avoiding an examination of what Jesus actually did given the absence of any eye witness report. Finally, even the harshest critics of the Jesus Seminar, would not deny that the sayings and parables ranked highest in terms of their probability of originating with Jesus, are not the words of Jesus.

If nothing else, by their painstaking evaluation, the participants in the Jesus Seminar have turned the spotlight on the wisdom teachings of Jesus. By highlighting these and comparing them to the words of other Jesus-like Yoga masters, the Siddhas, anyone can gain fresh insights into the truth lying there in. This is my primary purpose in writing this book. Spirituality relies upon the intimate and very personal communion between the individual's own consciousness and a truth that lies beyond words. By reflecting on the paradoxical, mystical sayings and parables of Jesus, one's religion goes beyond any belief system and becomes Truth itself.

More work of the type done by the Jesus Seminar could certainly be done in future, but what was accomplished was a tremendous effort with remarkable results. I have also found that the findings are consistent with what I have found to be true in the study of the Siddha literature. As we will see in the chapter entitled "Early Christianity: the Formation of the Church and its Dogma," their findings are also consistent with what many other modern critical scholars have found, but not by all.

Were the Gospels Inerrant and Inspired by God?

Why did Jesus' disciples remember so little of what he said, or remember them so inaccurately? Before answering this question one must first address the issue of the alleged verbal inspiration and inerrancy of the Bible, which is the basic assumption which most Christians maintain. Christians generally believe that the Spirit dictated the Gospels without error, or at least inspired those who wrote them. If this is so, however, why is it that those who hold this view are unable to agree on the picture of Jesus found in those same Gospels? The Jesus Seminar asked the question:

"Why are there as many Jesuses as there are interpretations of writings taken to be divinely dictated?

The endless proliferation of views of Jesus on the part of those who claim infallibility for the documents erodes confidence in that theological point of view and in the devotion to the Bible it supports. An inspired, or inerrant, set of Gospels seems to require an equally inspired interpreter or body of interpretation. Interpretation must be equally inspired if we are to be sure we have the right understanding of the inerrant but variously understood originals. There seems to be no other way to ascertain the truth. It is for this reason that some churches were moved to claim infallibility for their interpretation. And it is for the same reason that televangelists and other strident voices have made equally extravagant claims."[5]

Modern scholarship makes no such claims. It offers no more than tentative claims based on historical probability.

The question of infallibility begs another question: "Why, if God took such pains to preserve an inerrant text for posterity, did the spirit not provide for the preservation of original copies of the Gospels? It seems little enough to ask of a God who creates absolutely reliable reporters. In fact, we do not have original copies of any of the Gospels. We do not possess autographs of any of the books of the entire Bible. The oldest surviving copies of the Gospels date from about one hundred and seventy-five years after the death of Jesus, and no two copies are precisely alike. And handmade manuscripts have almost always been "corrected" here and there, often by more than one hand. Further, this gap of almost two centuries means that the original Greek (or Aramaic?) text was copied more than once, by hand, before reaching the stage in which it has come down to us. Even careful copyists make some mistakes, as every proofreader knows. So we will never be able to claim certain knowledge of exactly what the original text of any biblical writing was."[6]

The Church appears to have smothered the historical Jesus with a heavenly figure, as described in the Apostle's Creed: "... I believe in Jesus Christ, God's only Son, our Lord, who was conceived by the Holy Spirit, born of the Virgin Mary, suffered under Pontius Pilate, was crucified, died and was buried. He ascended into Heaven; He is seated at the right hand of the Father." Modern theologians and biblical scholars have both learned to distinguish the Jesus of history from the Christ of faith, the literary figure described in the canonical Gospels, and the heavenly, even mythical figure as portrayed in this Creed. Even many Roman Catholic scholars are participating in this research.

Two Portraits of Jesus: the Map of Relationships Between the Gospels

Modern historical research of the historical Jesus begins with the development of a critical edition of the Greek New Testament. Out of a mass of data gathered from over five thousand Greek manuscripts, some mere fragments, modern scholars have developed a composite text - a critical edition of the Greek New Testament. The dominance of the King James Version (1611) in the English speaking world, despite its many errors, delayed the development of the critical Greek text for 250 years. The discovery of the Codex Sinaiticus at St. Catherine's monastery in the Sinai Peninsula in 1844 prompted the first modern critical edition. More followed, as scholars pieced together its intricate history. The discoveries at Nag Hammadi and the Dead Sea scrolls assisted scholars in understanding the context for understanding Jesus and John the Baptist, as well as parts of the Old Testament. A complete copy of the Gospel of St Thomas found at Nag Hammadi, Egypt, in 1945, and several other Gospels, provided much significant information about the teachings of Jesus.

However, almost two centuries separate Jesus from the earliest surviving records of him. Scholars have therefore had to carefully analyze the network of complex relationships between the Gospels. The second pillar of historical scholarship, mentioned above, reveals that the two pictures painted by the three Synoptic Gospels and that of the Gospel of John cannot both be historically accurate. Jesus, the wise sage, the teller of parables and ethical teachings in Matthew, Mark and Luke, is "displaced in John by Jesus the revealer who has been sent from God to reveal who the Father is."[7]

This contrast is highlighted in the following table:

Two Portraits of Jesus

The Synoptic Gospels	*The Gospel of John*
Begins with John the Baptist	Begins with Creation
Birth and childhood stories	No birth or childhood stories
Jesus is baptized by John	Baptism of Jesus presupposed but not mentioned
Jesus speaks in parables and aphorisms	Jesus speaks in long, involved discourses
Jesus is a sage	Jesus is a philosopher and mystic
Jesus is an exorcist	Jesus performs no exorcisms
God's imperial rule is the theme of Jesus' teaching	Jesus Himself is the theme of His own teaching
Jesus has little to say about Himself	Jesus reflects extensively on his own mission and person
Jesus espouses the causes of the poor and oppressed	Jesus has little or nothing to say about the poor and oppressed
The public ministry lasts one year	The public ministry last three years
The temple incident is late	The temple incident is early
Jesus eats last supper with His disciples	Foot washing replaces last supper

8

The most important information regarding Jesus of Nazareth is derived from the three Synoptic Gospels, along with the Gospel of Thomas, which is considered by many scholars to be even older. The three Synoptic Gospels provide a "common view" of Jesus. Most scholars agree that Mark was written first, and that Matthew and Luke utilized Mark as their basis, and then added other materials. This conclusion is supported by the following arguments:

- "The agreement between Matthew and Luke begins where Mark begins and ends where Mark ends.
- Matthew reproduces about 90 percent of Mark, Luke about 50 percent. They often reproduce Mark in the same order. When they disagree, either Matthew or Luke supports the sequence in Mark.
- In those segments which the three have in common, (known as "the triple tradition") verbal agreement averages about 50 percent.
- In the triple tradition segments, Matthew and Mark often agree against Luke, and Luke and Mark often agree against Matthew, but Matthew and Luke only rarely agree against Mark."[9]

By comparing the three in columns, scholars can observe how Matthew and Luke edited Mark, in creating their own Gospel, according to their own perspective. So Mark is considered to be the fundamental source for narrative information about Jesus.

The fourth pillar of modern biblical scholarship rests upon the recognition that there are over two hundred verses where Matthew and Luke share a striking verbal agreement in passages where Mark offers nothing comparable. These are sayings and parables. This has lead scholars to believe that there once existed a source document, the so called "Q" which refers to *Quelle* (German – "source"). The discovery of the Gospel of Thomas reinforced the hypothesis that a Gospel could consist of only sayings, with no narratives. The hypothesis that Matthew and Luke utilized Mark and Q in creating their own texts is known as the two source theory, or double tradition.

After scholars extract the material from Q and Mark, there still remains a significant amount of material left over. Their sources have been referred to as M and L, unknown sources. These include some important parables, like that of the Good Samaritan, the prodigal son, the vineyard laborers, and the treasure and the pearl, which scholars believe originated with Jesus, and some of which have parallels in the Gospel of Thomas.

The Gospel of Thomas has no narratives, but consists of one hundred and fourteen sayings attributed to Jesus. It is a rich source of both new and comparative information. Thomas has forty seven parallels to Mark, forty to Q, seventeen to Matthew, four to Luke, and five to John. About sixty five sayings are unique to Thomas. These materials, which many scholars take to represent a tradition quite independent of the other Gospels, provide what scientists call a "control group," for the analysis of sayings and parables that appear in the other Gospels. So Thomas is a fifth independent source for the sayings and parables of Jesus. These are the major sources of information for the sayings and parables of Jesus.

Rules of Written Evidence

Over the past two hundred years, a large body of criteria or standards have been developed for evaluating the reliability of the evidence offered by the Gospels. These are known as "rules of written evidence" and enable scholars to evaluate what Jesus is reported to have said or done.[10]

All of the evidence provided by the written Gospels is "hearsay" evidence. Such evidence is inherently not very reliable, because it is secondhand evidence - someone told someone, who told someone else, who told someone else. Facts can become distorted in such a process, so scholars have to be very cautious in taking such evidence at face value. The authors of the four canonical Gospels are unknown. They were definitely not the four Apostles - Matthew, Mark, Luke and John. We do not know the names, or anything about the authors. In the case of the Gospel of Thomas the author is named as "Didymus Judas Thomas," revered as the twin brother of Jesus (so claimed by the Acts of Thomas, a third century work, as well as in the Syrian Church. His name, in Aramaic, means "twin"). However, like the authors of the canonical gospels, the author of the Gospel of Thomas was probably not the Apostle Thomas, but someone writing in his name, intending to express the "good news" as the disciple taught it.[11]

There are two categories of rules of evidence that scholars have developed. The first applies to written evidence, and applies to observations made about the "editorial habits" of Matthew and Luke as they make use of Mark and sayings in Gospel Q, as well as the direction in which the tradition developed. The second category pertains to rules of oral evidence. The Gospel of Thomas has also been influential in determining these rules.

The more important rules are summarized below:

- **Clustering and Contexting:** The authors of the Gospels grouped sayings and provided contexts for them, which usually affected their interpretation. These did not originate with Jesus. As it developed, the Gospel tradition tended to group sayings and parables into simple clusters at the oral stage, and into more extended complexes in the written stage. The Evangelists frequently relocated sayings and parables or invented new narrative contexts for them. These *chreia* (from the Greek *chreiodes*, "useful") stories consist of short anecdotes that climax in a witticism. This was done for several reasons: the Evangelists adopted and adapted the words of Jesus for their own needs, or because the original context of Jesus' witticisms was forgotten or unknown to the authors of the written Gospels. Generally, the sayings had circulated independently and orally, divorced from their context. This is evident when one compares them in the various Gospels.

- **Revision and Commentary:** The Evangelists frequently expanded sayings or parables, or provided them with an interpretive overlay or comment. They also often revised or edited sayings to make them conform to their own individual language, style or viewpoint.

- **False Attribution**: The Evangelists borrowed freely from common wisdom and coined their own sayings and parables, which they then attributed to Jesus. The concept of plagiarism was unknown in ancient times. Authors freely copied from earlier works without acknowledgement. Sages were collectors of free-floating proverbs and witticisms. Legendary sages like Solomon and Socrates attracted much such lore. For the early Christians, because Jesus was a legendary sage, it was proper to attribute the world's wisdom to him. The Greek Old Testament, called the *Septuagint*, was an especially popular source. The tendency of the Gospel writers, especially in the Gospel of Matthew, was to make the event fit the prophecies taken, and occasionally edited, from the Old Testament. For example, the scholars of the Jesus Seminar concluded that most of the words ascribed to Jesus, while he hung on the cross was not his: they were borrowed mostly from the Psalms and attributed to Jesus. The Evangelists also frequently attributed their own sayings to Jesus.

- **Difficult Sayings:** During the process of transmission, the early Christians frequently softened hard or harsh language in order to adapt them to their conditions of daily living. Variations in these difficult sayings often reveal the struggle of the early Christian community to interpret or adapt sayings to their own situation. A good example is the three variations of the "unforgivable sin:" blasphemy against the Holy Spirit (Mark 3.28-29, Luke 12:10 and Thomas 44: 1-3). All agree that it will not be forgiven, but differ as to what actually constituted blasphemy.

- **Christianizing Jesus:** Jesus was not the first Christian. However, He was often made to talk like a Christian by the anonymous writers of the Gospels. He was made to confess what Christians had come to believe. Sayings and parables expressed in "Christian" language are the creation of the early Christian preachers, known as the Evangelists or their Christian predecessors; for example, the famous "I am..." sayings in the Gospel of John. Sayings or parables that contrast with the language or viewpoint of the Gospel in which they are embedded reflect an older tradition (but not necessarily a tradition that originated from Jesus). The Christian community developed apologetic statements to defend its claims and sometimes attributed such statements to Jesus. Sayings and narratives that reflect knowledge of events that took place after Jesus' death are the creation of the Evangelists or the oral tradition before them. The contrast between Christian language or viewpoint and the language or viewpoint of Jesus is a very important clue to the real voice of Jesus, according to the Jesus Seminar scholars. The language and perspective of Jesus was distinctive, as was his style.

The Oral Tradition Prior to the Gospels and the Rules of Oral Evidence

Scholars are guided by the following basic rule when determining which sayings and parables can be attributed to Jesus:

"Only sayings and parables that can be traced back to the oral period, 30-50 C.E. can possibly have originated with Jesus."[12]

The oral period is defined, in broad terms, as the two decades extending from the death of Jesus to the composition of the first written Gospels, about 50 C.E. Sayings and stories continued to be circulated by word of mouth until well into the second century, given that few persons had access to the long scrolls of parchment, and even fewer could read or write. The first written Gospels were Sayings Gospel Q and probably an early version of the Gospel of Thomas. The Gospel of Mark was not composed until about 65 C.E.

Words that can be demonstrated to have been first formulated by the Gospel writers are eliminated from inclusion in those attributed to Jesus. Scholars search for two different kinds of proof. They look for evidence that particular formulations are characteristic of individual Evangelists or can only be understood in the social context of the emerging Christian movement. Or, they search for evidence that sayings and parables antedate the written Gospels.

The following four "rules of attestation" assisted the scholars of the Jesus Seminar to identify those sayings which can be assigned to the oral period with a high degree of probability:

1. Sayings or parables that are attested in two or more independent sources are older than the sources in which they are embedded.
2. Sayings or parables that are attested in two different contexts probably circulated independently at an earlier time.
3. The same or similar content attested in two or more different forms has had a life of its own and therefore may stem from old tradition.
4. Unwritten tradition that is captured by the written Gospels relatively late may preserve very old memories.[13]

Jesus taught his followers orally. He was an itinerant sage who dispensed wisdom wherever he went. His teachings were passed around by word of mouth by his disciples, improvising and adapting his most memorable sayings without reference to written records. The native tongue of Jesus was Aramaic, but his words have been preserved only in Greek. We do not know if he spoke Hebrew or Greek. If he did not speak Greek, then we must conclude that his exact words have been lost forever, with the exception of words like *Abba* (Aramaic - "Father"). (Recent archaeological evidence; however, reveals that Greek was widely known in the first century in Galilee.)

Knowledge of the transmission of oral tradition in many cultures has lead scholars to formulate the following three rules of oral evidence:

1. The oral memory best retains sayings and anecdotes that are short, provocative, memorable – and often repeated.
2. The most frequently recorded words of Jesus in the surviving Gospels take the form of aphorisms and parables.
3. The earliest layer of the Gospel tradition is made up of single aphorisms and parables that circulated by word of mouth prior to the written Gospels.[14]

Recent experiments with memory have led psychologists to conclude that most people forget the exact wording of a particular statement after only sixteen syllables, but that most are quite good at recalling the gist of what was heard or read. This has lead scholars to adopt the fourth rule:

4. Jesus' disciples remembered the core or gist of his sayings and parables, but not his precise words, except in rare cases.[15]

Those rare cases would include clichés and terms or phrases that Jesus employed on a regular basis. His followers would then repeat these too. Various leaders in the Jesus movement would then have started to develop their own independent streams of tradition, and these streams would eventually culminate in written Gospels like Thomas and the canonical Gospels. The surviving fragments of unknown Gospels indicate that there were once many Gospels. Twenty are known positively; there may have been many more. The Jesus tradition developed in many different directions simultaneously.

Under the storyteller's license to create, much of the incidental conversation of Jesus in anecdotes and narratives can be expected to be the creation of the storyteller. The scholars of the Jesus Seminar conclude that "We know that the Evangelists frequently ascribed words to Jesus to make him talk like a Christian, when in fact he was the precursor of a movement that took him as its cultic hero."[16]

The Distinctive Voice of Jesus

If the words of Jesus are to be isolated from those of other voices in the Gospels, the scholars of the Jesus Seminar had to make the following assumption:

Jesus' characteristic talk was distinctive – it can usually be distinguished from common lore. Otherwise it is futile to search for the authentic words of Jesus.

As scholars began to identify certain aphorisms and parables, because of their distinctiveness, as something Jesus probably said, the additional rules of evidence were formulated:

5. Jesus' saying and parables cut against the social and religious grain.

6. Sayings and parables surprise and shock; they characteristically call for a reversal of roles or frustrate ordinary, everyday expectations.
7. Jesus' sayings and parables are often characterized by exaggeration, humor, and paradox.
8. Jesus' images are concrete and vivid. His sayings and parables are customarily metaphorical and without explicit application.[17]

Those who heard Jesus must have wanted explanations, conclusions and explicit instructions. In return, Jesus gave them more questions, more stories with unclear references, more responses that waffle, shifting the decision back to the listeners. His style was not to give straightforward answers. Jesus never took away the power from people to decide how to behave or what to believe. Instead he gave them the responsibility to discover the truth for themselves.

The Unassertive Sage

Three additional rules of oral evidence have been formulated, relating to Jesus' lack of assertiveness:

9. Jesus does not as a rule initiate dialogue or debate, nor does he offer to cure people.
10. Jesus rarely makes pronouncements or speaks about himself in the first person.
11. Jesus makes no claim to be the Anointed, the Messiah.[18]

The modesty of Jesus, the sage is characteristic of the Hebrew prophets – Elijah and Elisha, for example, and of a holy man like Apollonius of Tyanan, a contemporary of Jesus, whose life is chronicled by Philostratus in the second century. Jesus did not initiate debates or controversies. He was passive until a question was put to him, or until he or his disciples were criticized. Even the Evangelists reflected vague memories of Jesus' unwillingness to speak about himself, or to assign himself heroic roles. In the synoptic accounts of his trial, Jesus remains stubbornly silent – for the most part. Jesus did not make claims about himself. The Christian community allowed its own triumphant faith to explode in confessions that were retrospectively attributed to Jesus, the authority figure. This culminated with the writing of the Gospel of John, in which Jesus does little but make claims for himself. For this reason, scholars regard John as alien to the real Jesus, the carpenter from Nazareth.

CHAPTER 2

Paradoxical Teachings of the God-men

In this chapter we will compare the teachings of Jesus with those of the Yoga Siddhas, as indicated in the Introduction. We will demonstrate the remarkable similarities between the authentic teachings of Jesus and those of the Yoga Siddhas. This comparison may shed light on the questions: "Who was Jesus?" "What were the mystical teachings of Jesus that he shared with selected disciples?" "Why did he teach as he did, in parables?" "Did he intentionally shock his listeners? And if so, why?" "Was Jesus a Guru?"

But before we do, we need to address some preliminary questions:

The Problem of Paradox: Was Jesus a Man or God?

What did Jesus really do, according to modern historical scholarship?

What is Yoga?

Who are the Yoga Siddhas?

What is the literature of the Yoga Siddhas?

The Problem of Paradox

As will be seen in the chapter on Early Christianity, the proto-Orthodox Christians succeeded in establishing their version of Christianity by enshrining it, in 493 A.D., in the Nicaean Creed - that Jesus Christ is truly God and truly man, without offering a logical resolution of the paradox of such an assertion. How can one be both infinite and finite? Divine and human? As Georg Feuerstein put the dilemma cogently: "If we can learn anything from the centuries of scholastic exertions in Christianity, it is that in order to understand the divinity of the adept, who is human, we must come to terms with the inherent paradox of the enlightened being."[1]

In the Gospels of Matthew, Mark and Luke, Jesus made no special claims about Himself. He did not claim to be the "Anointed one," the Christ, the Messiah. So who was he? Christianity developed out of various attempts to answer this question.

Westerners in particular have a problem with paradox. The languages of Greek, English and Hebrew, which are the foundation of the Western view of the world, are dualistic languages. So we think and speak in terms like "right" and "wrong," "high" and "low," "sacred" and "profane," "true" and "false," and "God" and "human." These terms are mutually exclusive, so when something exhibits both, it is a paradox, which confounds our patterns of thinking about and seeing reality.

The fact that what Jesus said was translated into Greek and then into English makes it even more difficult to conceive of "both" when considering the vision of the God-man. The God-man sees the transcendental One amidst the many. He sees the "Kingdom of Heaven" here, within and without. How to express this in a dualistic language? Metaphor, paradox, parables, parody all serve to jolt the listener out of their dualistic thinking. They challenge the listeners to go beyond words, logic and creeds and into a new perspective, and then into silence where pure consciousness reigns.

What Did Jesus Really Do, According to Modern Historical Research?

We can examine the consensus about what Jesus said and what he did not say. But with regards to what Jesus did, scholars have come to a broad consensus that we do not know, except that he was an itinerant teacher of wisdom who probably lived at the beginning of the Christian era and taught some original parables and aphorisms in the region of ancient Judea, Samaria and Galilee. We do not know the circumstances of his birth, what happened during the so-called missing years, whether he performed miracles, or even whether he was crucified, entombed, resurrected and ascended into heaven, as the Gospels narrate.

There are no eyewitness accounts. There are no historical documents that corroborate any of the claims made in the Gospels. We cannot know what Jesus really did with any degree of assurance even remotely approaching the certainties we have about what Jesus really taught. For the same reason, we cannot know what the Yoga Siddhas did with any degree of assurance for rarely did they write about themselves. What was written about what they did were sometimes from eye witness reports, but cannot be authenticated. What is interesting and important to consider is that the Siddhas wrote, hundreds of years before Jesus was born, many of the same Truths of which Jesus spoke. In addition they taught in a similar manner. That the Siddhas lived and taught wisdom is certain; exactly what they did, as far as miracles are concerned is not.

There is some evidence although not conclusive that Jesus went to India before his ministry, during the so-called missing years and again after his crucifixion. Holger Kersten, in his book *Jesus Lived in India*, went about as far as anyone could to report on this evidence. However, we do not need to determine whether Jesus lived in India or not to gain insights into who he was and what he taught. His teaching and mission can be satisfactorily explained on the basis of Judaism and the tendency to reconcile differing belief systems during the Age of his life. But we can directly compare the wisdom attributed to Jesus and the manner of his teaching with the wisdom and teaching style of the sages or Siddhas of Yoga, in India.

As Georg Feuerstein wrote: "We need not assume that he was personally initiated into, or even informed about, any Indian yogic teachings. Even if he was exposed to migrant Indian scholars with some knowledge of Yoga, his teachings and mission can be satisfactorily explained on the basis of Judaism and the syncretistic philosophical movements at work during his era. In other words, it was home grown. The New Age notion of Jesus as a full-fledged yogin trained in the Himalayas appears to be due to historical myopia. Therefore we may speak about his teaching as a form of Yoga only by way of comparison."[2]

What is Yoga?

This question needs to be answered before many Christians will even begin to appreciate a comparison between the historical teachings of Jesus and those of the Yoga Siddhas.

Yoga is not a religion; however it could be viewed to be the practical side of all religions. Religions are, by definition, systems of belief, which trace their origins to humans who were inspired to share their wisdom or divine realizations. To practice Yoga one needs no belief in any religion; one must only be open to spirituality, following the curve of expanding consciousness to its origin, believing that one can transform oneself.

While many Yoga masters have been historically associated with India's great religions: Hinduism, Buddhism, Jainism and Sikhism, there is no agreement between these religions with regards to the reality of deities, karma and reincarnation. Yoga emphasizes no philosophical or theological beliefs, but practical experimentation, verification, and realization. It is therefore scientific in that it proposes hypotheses (the techniques of *Yoga*), testing (practice) and recording of experiences and comparison with other practitioners, just as modern scientists do. But it is also an art, in that it requires practice and skill to overcome one's human nature, which resists change due to deep seated habit patterns. Yoga emphasizes direct, personal experience or realization over any conceptual description of reality.

There are various forms of Yoga, which address the various levels of our human being:

- Hatha Yoga: physical postures, muscular locks and *mudras* (symbolic gestures) which heal, energize and relax the physical body, strengthen the nervous system, and prepare one for breathing and meditation exercises. This is the most popular form in the West, which has discovered its beneficial effects in controlling stress.
- Pranayama: breathing exercises that utilize awareness in order to energize and strengthen the nervous system, calm the mind, and balance the function of both hemispheres of the brain. *Kundalini Yoga* emphasizes those pranayama, which circulate vital energy through subtle psycho-energetic centers known as *chakras*, and which awaken potential spiritual energy, known as *kundalini*.
- Dhyana (chan, zen) or meditation: the scientific art of concentrating and mastering the mind; the cultivation of powerful awareness, which can transcend the ordinary ego perspective.
- Mantra Yoga: the use of potent sound syllables to awaken the intellect and intuition, to purify the subconscious, to awaken the *chakras* and to develop virtuous qualities.
- Bhakti Yoga: the cultivation of love and aspiration for the Divine through devotional activities.

While we do not have any evidence that Jesus practiced yogic methods, there, are however, strong indications in his teachings that he practiced some forms of meditation and certainly prayer and devotional activities, what we may refer to as Bhakti Yoga. His aspiration for the Divine was profound and was consistently demonstrated in his simplicity, humility, preaching and compassionate acts toward the sick and infirm. Intense devotion to God, humility, non-harming and compassion for others are also demonstrated in the lives of the Yoga Siddhas.

Yoga as a Philosophy

Yoga is considered to be one of the six major systems of orthodox Indian philosophy, known as *darshanas* or perspectives on the creation and laws of the Universe. It derives from two older systems, *Samkhya* and *Vedanta*. The *darshans* are the expressions of the *Siddhas* and *Rishis*. Each *darshan* has a *Siddha* to whom it is attributed. Each *darshan* has *sutras*, initial "threads" that formed a beginning to the development of the system. The methods and perceptions of each intertwine.

Samkhya: the oldest *darshana,* is associated with the sage Kapila and the *Samkhya-Sutras*. The *Bhagavad-Gita* also expounds *Samkhya*. For Krishna, Yoga and *samkhya* are equivalent. It includes twenty-four principles or constituents of nature (*tattvas)*, which analyze how the One is seen as subject and object and how the objective reality manifests as the many in nature. The twenty four *tattvas* are: the five elements (earth, water, fire, air, ether or space), the five sense essences (seeing, hearing, smelling, tasting, touching), the five organs of cognition (eyes, ears, nose, tongue, skin), the five organs of action (feet, hands, voice, digestion, reproduction), mind, intellect, consciousness and ego. Individual souls are real, but kept from liberation from the world by ignorance of their true identity. It says that matter and the universe are real and not an illusion, yet the goal of existence is liberation (*moksha*) from it. It is dualistic: nature versus consciousness and object versus subject. It underlies Yoga, *Vedanta, Tantra* and other *darshanas*. Initially it could have been considered atheistic, but evolved to include subtle divine principles or attributes of a Supreme God.

Vedanta: is associated with sage Vyasa and is the end of the *Vedas*, the oldest spiritual texts of India, comprising 200 odd commentaries on them known as the *Upanishads*. *Veda* means knowledge. Its essence is the eternal principle of God (*Brahman)*, and that nothing exists outside God (*Brahman)*. It declares that there is oneness to all things. It is non-dualistic – monistic (belief in One pervasive unified whole), not theistic (belief in a personal creator God, who rules the world). While it contains the principles or *tattvas* of *Samkhya*, they are due only to the One Brahman. Their separate existence is felt due to ignorance of the True Reality (*avidya)* underlying the objective illusion (*maya)*.

The individual has five sheaths or bodies, through which the world *(maya)* influences us. Its' concepts of our human nature are the physical body or sheath *(kosha)*, the vital or subtle energy body which is the seat of the emotions and which animates the physical body, the mental body of the senses, imagination, and memory, the intellectual body of reason and inspiration, and the most sublime soul *(atman)*, the spiritual self and pure consciousness. *Atman* is ultimately *Brahman*, as the individual soul *(atman)* is none other than the One Supreme Soul, shared by all. The nature of Brahman is Absolute being, Absolute consciousness and Absolute bliss *(satchidananda)*.

Yoga Darshan: is associated with Patanjali and his *Yoga Sutras*. It refers to the Lord of Yoga as *Ishvara* (literally, *Siva*, meaning one's own special Self) twelve times, and it says that through Ashtanga and Kriya Yogas one can know the Lord. In a state of cognitive absorption or *samadhi* when the individual enters a transcendental state of consciousness, in the deepest meditation, taking nourishment directly from cosmic energy through a stream above the head, rather than through breathing, when the mind, heart and senses shut down and yet life is retained. In this state one can know the Lord. This state of samadhi, which unites one with God and grants true wisdom takes the middle position between *Samkhya's* dualism and *Vedanta's* non-dualism. It is based in both of them. It is theistic and dualistic.

Yoga is experiential and experimental. It insists that the transcendental state of *Samadhi* (cognitive absorption) is necessary for realization of the Self and that mere rational knowledge will never allow one to transcend the ego-self. Self-realization is only accessible through intensive personal application to the practices of Yoga. Like *Samkhya,* it has as its objective liberation or *moksha*, wherein one identifies wholly with the Self, and nevermore with the fluctuations of the mind. It also shares *Vedanta's* supreme goal of merging the individual Self with the Absolute. It is both practical and theoretical.

Classical *Yoga,* as expounded by the Siddha Patanjali, (200 C.E.) includes the methods of Astanga (eight limbed) Yoga: social ethical restraints, and personal observances, postures, breath control, sense control, concentration, meditation and cognitive absorption. It aims to first reduce and then eliminate the causes of human suffering. It declares that through Kriya Yoga, including intense practice, self-study and surrender to the Lord, the causes of suffering are gradually eliminated and Self-realization is attained. According to it, the five causes of human suffering are ignorance, egoism, attachment, aversion, and clinging to life. The practices of Yoga allow one to become aware of, understand, organize, and even to control, the twenty-four principles of nature (*tattvas*). This occurs progressively as one realizes one's unity with the All. One comes to understand that unity is as strong a principle in nature as is division. Unity is in fact, the master principle of which diversity is a sub-component.

Who Are the Yoga Siddhas?

There are several usages of the term *Siddha*. The most common use of the term is to describe a "perfected being," or "one who has become one with God," or "one who has realized the non-duality of their psyche, or individual soul's consciousness and the consciousness of the Lord," or "an adept yogin, who possesses specific psychic or supernatural powers, known as *siddhis*." The eight categories of *siddhis* are as follows:

1. *Anima:* the ability to become as minute as an atom.
2. *Mahima:* the ability to expand infinitely.
3. *Laghima:* levitation, or the ability to float through the air.
4. *Garima:* the ability to reach everywhere.
5. *Prakamya:* a freedom of will, or the ability to overcome natural obstacles.
6. *Isitva:* the ability to create or control.
7. *Vasitva:* domination over the entire creation.

8. *Kamavasayitva:* the gift of wish fulfillment, or the ability to attain everything desired or to attain the stage of desirelessness.

We may begin to gain some understanding of who the Siddhas are by comparing and contrasting them with more familiar terms of reference. The Yoga Siddhas are mystics, but they are also much more. The word "mystic" is derived from the Greek word *muein,* which means to close the lips and eyes. However, these two outward indications of mystical experience only suggest the inner state of the mystic, wherein one perceives the oneness of everything, transcending the ordinary subject versus object duality of the ordinary mind.

In the ordinary state of consciousness, one fails to perceive the underlying reality, that which is constant, eternal and infinite; the mind, instead, contracts around objects experienced through the five senses, thoughts, memories or emotions. To use an analogy, one sees only the waves on the surface of the ocean. The mystic, however, not only sees the entire ocean, but plunges into it, merging with it in transcendental bliss. While for the mystic, the comings and goings of experiences, like waves on the surface of the ocean, are real, they pale in significance in comparison with the mystic's insight into the one Being, Consciousness and Bliss, the joy of unity.

The term "mystic," furthermore, is generally limited to only the first stages of spiritual development, at least in Western literature. The spirit has no form, and so since the time of the Renaissance, the study of mysticism has been largely supplanted in the West by the study of Nature, objective reality, the other side of the subject-object coin. However, many scientists who are probing the origins of objective reality have come to appreciate the significance of mysticism in the modern era. Einstein referred to the essence of mysticism as the finest thing we can experience. It is the fundamental emotion at the roots of science. It may be defined as "consummation... an instantaneous, intuitive insight loaded with the feeling that it is not accessible to common sense, rational training or learning."[3]

When Einstein was accused of plagiarism in the origin of his famous theory of relativity, he wrote in his defense that his discovery of it was not deduced through a rational process of deduction, but that it arose within him as a spontaneous flash of insight. Such insight characterizes the mystics' realizations.

When mystical communion with the spiritual dimension of life becomes facile and the norm, we may refer to the mystic as a "saint." The ordinary egoistic perspective of a saint is replaced at least in part, by an awareness of the Presence of the Divine. Egoism is the habit of identifying with the body, its sensations, the emotions and the movements of the mind. As we let go of this false identification, the background, which is pure consciousness, becomes the foreground. One surrenders the ordinary ego perspective ("I am the body," or "I am thinking") to that of the soul ("I am") or that of the Witness. The Witness does not do or think or feel anything. It is the awareness, itself. The Witness simply is, and watches things get done, watches thoughts, sensations and feelings come and go. The soul or Witness has no form. It is pure consciousness, the subject. The mind and nature are objects. The soul perceives all of this coming and going as emanating from and disappearing into the One, an infinite, eternal, Nameless Supreme Being. This is not an intellectual or theological affirmation, but an intensely personal, even ecstatic perspective.

However, if the mystic's surrender or communion is limited to the spiritual plane of reality only, he may still be bound by a need to make philosophical or theological distinctions until he begins to surrender his ego in the intellectual plane. A Christian mystic may refer to "my belief" or "my faith" and a Buddhist mystic may say "I think" or refer to other word symbols. A Christian mystic may seek to attribute his or her insights to Jesus, or to this Christian faith. A Buddhist may use word symbols as he seeks to translate his experience of mystical oneness into forms that can be communicated. As the surrender deepens however, the "I" and the "mine" are gradually let go of, the ego is dissolved and Silent Awareness pervades all one thinks, says and does. No more can divided units of mind and intellect struggle with one another. There is no more "my" and "yours" to compel or influence or resist; there is no need to gather information.

One becomes a sage in the intellectual plane of existence when one is able to enter a state of identification through *samadhi* (cognitive absorption) in communion with any subject one contemplates. In that state one can access any subject with intimate familiarity because one has transcended the subject/object barrier. One is in a state of communion with the object.

The ego still lingers however, until the surrender encompasses all planes of existence. There is always the risk of a fall, and desire, aversion, clinging to life can still create suffering. As Saint Augustine put it: "Lord, help me to surrender, but not yet." That is, part of our lower human nature, in particular the mental plane, the seat of fantasy and desires, and the vital plane, the seat of the emotions, resists the transformation which surrender entails. As the mystic's surrender deepens still further and embrace the mental plane, wherein lies the five senses, one becomes a Siddha, manifesting siddhis (divine powers), beginning with clairvoyance - the ability to see things at a distance in time or space, or clairaudience - the subtle sense of hearing, or clairsentience - the subtle sense of feeling. One may make prophecies, manifest the capacity to heal the sick, and know the past of others by intuitive insight, as one can enter into deep states of communion with the past, future, or any aspect of an object upon which one concentrates.

A few rare Siddhas succeed in surrendering their ego at the level of the vital plane of existence. There they become Maha Siddhas or great Siddhas, capable of manifesting *siddhis* or powers, which involve nature itself. This may include materialization of objects, levitation, control of the weather, wish fulfillment and invisibility. While they have lived principally in India, Tibet, China, and southeast Asia, by their own accounts, the Siddhas have traveled all over the world.[4] We have examples of many such *Siddhas* in the twentieth century, for example: in Paramahansa Yogananda's *Autobiography of a Yogi, Miracles of Love,* the story of Neem Karoli Baba, *Living with Himalayan Masters,* by Swami Rama, *Maharaj: a biography of Shriman Tapasviji Maharaj, a Mahatma who lived for 185 years,* by T.S. Anantha Murthy, *Arut Perum Jothi and the Deathless Body* about Ramalinga Swamigal by by T. R. Thulasiram and *Sri Aurobindo: the Adventure of Consciousness,* by Satprem. These accounts demonstrate that the reported miracles of Jesus were not unique. The accounts, by eye witnesses are often as humorous as they are moving.

Neem Karoli Baba, was named, for example, after a village where he performed a miracle early in the twentieth century. Prior to this, he was known as "Well Baba" by villagers in the Garwhal Himalayas because he spent many years in intensive Yoga practice (*tapas*) at the bottom of a well. Because of the tremendous heat produced in his physical body due to his austerities, it was the only place he could keep sufficiently cool! One day, he boarded a train. When asked by the train conductor to produce his ticket for verification, he said that he had none. The conductor forced him off the train at the next stop, a village named after the "Neem" tree, "Neem Karoli." But when the train's engineer tried to make the train depart, it would not move. Hours passed. The engineer could find no reason to explain why the train would not move. Everyone was becoming impatient. Then one of the passengers spotted the old Baba sitting on the platform by the train and thought, perhaps the train will not move because the conductor forced the old Baba off the train? Several passengers then scolded and pressured the conductor to put the old Baba back onto the train. As soon as he did, the train departed. Thereafter he was known as "Neem Karoli Baba."

Siddhas like Neem Karoli Baba also healed the sick and dying, as Jesus did, but with a sense of humor! One day, Neem Karoli Baba was sitting in a barber's chair, with shaving cream on his face when a young man ran into the barber's shop, crying. He pleaded with Neem Karoli Baba to come and help his relative, who was at home deathly ill in bed, over fifty miles away. Neem Karoli Baba became completely motionless. At about this same time, it was subsequently reported by the dying man's relatives sitting by his bedside, Neem Karoli Baba suddenly ran into the room, with shaving cream on his face, and healed the dying man.

A few rare *Siddhas* are able to surrender their egos at the level of the physical plane. Even for the most serious of Yogis, this is difficult to conceive of, if one remains tied to the old paradigm of opposition between spirit/consciousness and the body and the world. What I am speaking of, is such an advanced stage of ego purification, that the cells of the physical body surrender their limited agenda of metabolism and become subject to the direction of ones' greatly expanded consciousness. The physical body glowing with the light of this consciousness becomes impervious to disease and death.

The Siddha Patanjali tells us that until the old habits of identifying with the body and mind are completely uprooted, by repeatedly returning to the source of consciousness, the ego is still able to delude at times the saint or Siddha. They may for example, use their powers to attract public attention. However, once the surrender occurs even at the physical level, the ego is banished forever. One is literally "nothing special," because one is only identified with That, which permeates everything: pure consciousness. This appears to have been the state of Jesus the Christ. Certain Siddhas through the ages have reached this state and these Siddhas placed no emphasis or importance on their person, their powers, their biography, or their motions- because those were not "theirs." These enlightened beings were instruments of the Divine force and Light and all action and rest that moved through them were due to that Divine Power. It is therefore no coincidence that we know with so little certainty what Jesus and other Siddhas did, or what were the details of their *personal* lives, but we do know their wisdom teachings. It is the wisdom they attained, which they have taken pains to leave for us. It is this Christ-consciousness, this wisdom, this experience of the ultimate Reality that they considered to be of utmost importance, because it will show us the way back to the "Kingdom of Heaven."

The Siddha may be called upon to remain in the same physical body for some indefinite period of time, or even to transmigrate into another body or to dematerialize, or to ascend as Jesus did, or to be in more than one, visible body at the same period of time, in two separate places. There is the well-documented example of Ramalinga Swamigal, of the late nineteenth century, whose body cast no shadow in the sun, whose body could not be harmed, or photographed, despite repeated attempts when he posed with a group before expert photographers, and whose body disappeared from the earth, quite dramatically, in a flash of violet light. Since then, Ramalinga Swamigal has been reported to have reappeared on occasions to assist devotees in need. Children and devotees in southern India to this day continue to sing many of the more than forty thousand poems and songs he wrote, extolling the path of "supreme grace light." We also have the example of Kriya Babaji, described in the *Autobiography of a Yogi*, and *The Voice of Babaji: A Triology of Kriya Yoga*, and that of the Siddhas Agastyar, Boganathar and Sri Aurobindo, who left detailed accounts of their own process of surrendering at the level of the physical body and various forms of immortality. As Mircea Eliade states: the *Siddha*s are those "who understood liberation as the conquest of immortality."[5]

Once this process of surrender of the ego fully embraces the intellectual plane of existence, the mystic is no longer apt to emphasize the authority of scriptures. One's own experience becomes the ultimate authority of one's truth. The Siddha is a free thinker and a revolutionary who refuses to allow himself to be carried away by any dogma, scripture or ritual.[6] The Siddha is a radical in the true sense of the term, for he has personally gone to the "root" of things, and finding the truth there can no longer be bound by the injunctions of scriptures.

Sectarian affiliation has no importance for Siddhas. They feel at ease among persons of all faiths. Their approach towards truth is to first experience it in *samadhi*, the mystical communion of cognitive absorption, and then to gradually surrender to it completely until it becomes their constant state of consciousness in the state of enlightenment. Their approach does not include attempts to build systems of philosophy or to construct religious belief systems. The Siddhas' poems show no trace of shared opinions or collective thinking; theirs is an "open philosophy" in which all expressions of truth were valued. Their poems and songs do not preach any doctrines; they only suggest a direction by which aspiration for a direct, intuitive, personal and profound realization of the Divine truth may be realized.

The *Siddhas,* however, used a forceful, vernacular language designed to shock people out of their conventional morality and egoistic delusion. They used the common language of the people, rather than the elitist Sanskrit, in order to reach their listeners. They urged their listeners to rebel against pretentious, empty orthodox beliefs and practices, including temple worship and rituals, caste, and petitionery prayers.

Those who attribute ultimate authority to scriptures, traditions, rituals and temple worship on the other hand, including the Brahmins and *Vedic* scholars and priests, usually misunderstood the Siddhas. They criticized, even ridiculed the Siddhas for their common language and irreverence for tradition. Their reaction was not unlike that of the Christian proto-Orthodox towards the Christian Gnostics and other lost Christianities. The Gnostics and the Siddhas both emphasized an inner knowing, the result of esoteric, personal experience and practices involving initiation of those who had become worthy. The Yoga Siddhas belong to a non-conformist "counter-tradition," which means not "that which opposes tradition," but "the tradition which opposes," the established order.[7]

The Yoga Siddhas, for example, challenged many of the accepted beliefs and practices of Hindu society and thought. Consequently many people thought they were Buddhists in disguise, as Buddhists also strongly criticized the doctrines and practices of the Hindus. Buddha, of course was not a Buddhist. Later, as Buddhism itself became a religion, Buddha became an object of worship, just as Jesus did. A comparison of Tibetan Buddhism reveals that Lord Siva was replaced by Buddha as the central object of worship, but that many of the practices and aspirations are very similar. Advanced Tibetan Buddhists are acknowledged as being Yoga Siddhas as well.

What is the Literature of the Yoga Siddhas?

The writings of the Yoga Siddhas spans many centuries and represents a variety of views not crystallized into any well defined doctrines. One therefore cannot explain their wisdom teachings in terms of one philosophy or even one historical line of development.

Furthermore, most of the Yoga Siddha literature remains unpublished, particularly that of southern India, written in the language of Tamil. Their works were not well preserved by the institutions which would normally have done so - the temples for example, which were controlled by the Brahmins. There are thousands of palm leaf manuscripts in Tamil Nadu, the southern most state of India. These are written on palm leaves, which have a life of three to four hundred years, so existing manuscripts are copies of copies of copies going back to the first centuries of the common Christian era.

Since the year 2000, the Yoga Siddha Research Project has succeeded in preserving over one thousand of these manuscripts. It has also transcribed a large number of these into a useful modern form of Tamil and selected samples of these for translation and commentary in six publications to date.

As a result of these studies the following observations can be made in general about the writings of the Tamil Yoga Siddhas:

- We are at an early stage in the study of this literature. Before extensive comparisons and analysis can be made, all of the existing manuscripts must be preserved and critically evaluated.
- There is a continuing process of corruption and interpolation in the Siddha texts. Later editions have a tendency to tamper with original works.
- The basic source of the Tamil Siddha poetry and philosophy is the vernacular of the people. Much of what we have today of Siddha poetry has been handed down in the form of oral transmission from one generation to another. To facilitate oral transmission, the Siddhas used only common words spoken by ordinary people - often with crude, sometimes offensive colloquial expressions. This produces a powerful effect on the reader of these poems. This is not unlike the "sayings" of Jesus, which were the first things to be written down eventually by early Christians.
- There are at least two levels of meaning expressed by the Siddha's poetry: the outer or superficial and the esoteric or symbolic. Only

the latter can be understood by the initiate, who is given the means to reflect deeply and to understand the hidden meaning. Because it reflects the inner experience of the Siddha, it is often difficult to comprehend unless one can replicate that inner experience within oneself. The poetry also draws upon a rich variety of sources: folklore, and the sacred literature known as the *Tantras,* the *Vedas,* and the *Agamas*; so one must consider all of these when seeking to understand the poetry. Understanding it requires an awareness of the total religious and philosophical structures infused into it.[8] One must enter deep states of meditation wherein each verse serves as a key for the initiate, opening a door to high truths and insight. The disciples of Jesus must have had similar difficulty in understanding His teachings, which expressed His personal insights and experience, enriched by the rich tapestry of ancient Judaism. Most of them were ordinary uneducated laborers, who had been with him for a relatively short period, not more than a year.

- Much of the Siddha poetry makes use of twilight language (*sandhya bhasa*) a symbolic, secret language, the intention of which was to deliberately obscure the hidden meaning from the uninitiated. In doing so, it protected the sacred from being profaned by the ignorant. The use of this language has been a source of mistrust of the Siddha's teachings by exponents of other systems of philosophy and religion in India. Opponents of the Siddhas' teachings, not unlike the proto-Orthodox Christians' attacks on the Christian Gnostics, have criticized the Siddhas' intentionally obscure and symbolic language. This lack of regard and understanding by the orthodox Hindus and their temples, monasteries and libraries has contributed to the paucity of study and understanding of the Siddhas' teachings. Scholars have avoided the Siddha literature because it is so difficult to decipher.

The twilight language is characterized by a deceptive simplicity. The highest teachings are often expressed in the lowest forms of expression. It makes free use of paradox, wordplay, typology, metaphors, numerals and alphabet symbolism to express a sublime reality hidden behind words and symbols. The paradoxical expressions are usually only accessible to understanding by the initiated - the techniques gained during initiation permitting them to access the deeper truths.[9] For example:

"Watch out for the blossoming circle

And the oil beneath; that is the flame.

As you hold on without losing your fervor,

There appears He, as the moon".

- Samadhi-12, verse 8 by the Siddha Cattaimuni[10]

This verse is filled with twilight language. When one reaches the state of *samadhi* one must not think that the final goal has been reached. Without losing fervor, one must maintain the state and perceive the Lord, represented by the "moon." The "oil" is a metaphor for the Lord, who dwells within, unperceived, like the oil, which dwells inside the seed. The blossoming circle is the crown *chakra*. The flame is the source of light, just as the Lord is the source of consciousness. It is the Lord Himself, which fuels the fire of aspiration.

Here is another example:

"Let me speak. Entwining intelligence with silence

Remain firm as long as mind can hold.

I shall speak, though it is not easy, my son!

See within this the welding and the division.

If the base of intelligence is found

The physical body becomes one of camphor,

As Siva comes to reside in this temple

He gives gathered food for us to eat".

- *Cutta Jnanam*-16, verse 6 by the *Siddha* Konganavar[11]

Here the Siddha is attempting to describe an experiential methodology. Intelligence has innumerable things to think about. It must be joined with silence to avoid wastage and then plunged into meditation. Then the division of the mind is overcome and one finds the base from which flowers our intelligence. This prepares one for illumination. The Lord comes and feeds the body with spiritual illumination. Camphor is a symbol of the divinized body, which will leave no trace of its former physical presence after it is illumined.by God consciousness. Many of the great saints including Ramalinga wre reported to have a physical body which could cast no shadow. Sri Aurobindo referred to this as the descent of the supramental.

The poems of the Siddhas have "the advantage of precision, concentration, secrecy, and mystery in that their symbols are objective shortcuts to subjective states of bliss."[12] The highly suggestive poetry, when reflected upon deeply, leads the reader into experience of spiritual truths which are inexpressible. By entering deep states of meditation while reflecting upon them, the initiate can use them as one would use a key to open a door lock, and thereby gain access to their hidden meaning. The Siddha Tirumular indicated that each verse he wrote was the fruit of one year of contemplation, a summary so to speak. To know their meaning requires a similar effort in deep reflection.

Similarities Between Jesus, the Yoga Siddhas and their Teachings

A comparison of the teachings of Jesus and those of the Siddhas reveals remarkable similarities:

1. Manner of teaching: Jesus taught in parables, metaphor, paradox, and parody, conveying profound teachings in a way that illiterate listeners could easily understand and remember. He was profoundly iconoclastic, and sought to move, even shock his listeners to realize the spirit, not the letter of the Jewish law and worship practices. The Yoga Siddhas taught in the form of poems, in the language of the illiterate people, in a way that they could easily understand, memorize and recall. Their language was also paradoxical and intended to shock the listener out of conventional perspectives.

Several layers of meaning can be attributed to both the sayings of Jesus and the poems of the Siddhas. The deepest layers can be understood only by the initiate - those who have been taught by a spiritual master how to access the inner reality through such practices as meditation and silence. The Gnostic Christians insisted that they had received such initiations; there are authentic Biblical references to Jesus giving such initiations to Paul, Judas and Thomas.

2. Condemnation of religious authorities over temple worship: Jesus severely condemned the Pharisees and the merchants in the temple, physically assaulting their shops. When challenged by the Pharisees on what authority did he speak, he replied: "I shall destroy this temple, and within three days, raise it up!" His resurrection from the cross proved his point, that the real temple is within ourselves.

The Yoga Siddhas also condemned emphasis on temple worship and idol worship. Nowhere in any of their writings do they sing in praise of any of the popular Hindu deities or images of God. They taught that the true temple of God is the human body, and that only by a process of inner purification can one come to know the Lord. All the orthodox systems suspected the Siddhas because they advocated the theory that one can attain *moksa* (freedom) while still within the body. Their aim was perfection of the body (*kaya-siddhi*).

3. Becoming "perfect": The term Siddha means one who has attained "perfection." God-realization in a diseased body was not something they could consider "perfection." They would agree with Jesus' admonition: "Be ye Perfect" and they sought after this through progressive purification at all levels of their being: becoming saints in the spiritual plane of existence in divine communion; becoming sages in the intellectual plane, conversant with all subjects by direct intuitive perception; becoming Siddhas with psychic powers in the mental plane; Maha Siddhas or adepts with even greater powers such as materialization and control over natural forces in the vital plane; and in a few cases, surrendering the ego perspective completely to the Divinity even in the cells of the physical body, attaining physical immortality. The Siddhas' teachings and poems

have not gained the official sanction from the orthodox elites and educated castes of India, but are popular among the masses.

4. Forgiveness: Forgiveness was one of Jesus' principal teachings, such as in the Lord's Prayer (Matthew 6.12), and in Luke 6.37: "Forgive and you will be forgiven." The Siddhas taught how to "detach" from the influence of subconscious tendencies, (*samskaras),* which collectively are referred to as karma, that is, the consequences of actions, words and thoughts. Forgiveness and dispassion (*vairagya*) are synonymous at a deep level of understanding, and are central to both the teachings of Jesus and Siddhas.

Forgiveness is a special case of dispassion, or detachment, as it is practiced in Yoga. When one forgives, one lets go of resentment, judgment, hurt, and every other thought or feeling that may stem from one's reaction to what someone else has said or done. This letting go, or detachment depends upon the recognition that one is not the thoughts and feelings. "We will be forgiven" means that we will dissolve the karmic habit of reacting out of confusion as to who we are, and realize our pristine true Self. When we fail to forgive, on the other hand, we become absorbed in the thoughts and feelings and lose awareness of our true Self. This brings more suffering. We also reinforce further the *samskara* or habit which produced our reaction. The development of detachment is the principle method of Patanjali's Kriya Yoga, as stated in his Yoga Sutra I.12: "By constant practice and with detachment (arises) the cessation of identifying with the fluctuations of consciousness."

5. God and the soul: they are not two: Both Jesus and the Siddhas used a dualistic philosophical approach to teach. With reference to themselves and God, the Siddhas emphasized: "they are not two," and the individual soul (jiva) is becoming "the Lord." Philosophically, this is known as "monistic theism," and represents a blending of non-dualistic monism and dualistic theism. The soul and God are both real and distinct, yet they are one. Jesus sometimes distinguished himself from the Lord, whom he called "the Father," and at other times said things like "I am my Father are one." This monistic theism can be best understood with the use of a metaphor: the individual soul is like the wave on the surface of

the ocean, part and particle with the ocean, yet, for a time, distinct. It originates from the ocean, and returns to it. However, the soul is not equivalent to God. The Siddhas taught that the Lord has functions, which the soul does not have: creation, preservation, destruction, obscuration and grace.

6. God is love: Jesus taught that the Lord, whom he referred to as the Father, not only exists, but that He loves you. He also taught that to know Him, one must overcome egoism and attachment to the things of this world. The Siddhas taught that the Lord is love (*anbu Sivam*). They cultivated intense aspiration for surrender, and merging with the Lord in deep states of ecstasy. Their poetry, often written in the first person, expressed their heartfelt devotion for the Lord. From the religious perspective they advocated monotheism. Their worship, however, was not in temples, but within themselves. They practiced internal worship through meditation and Kundalini Yoga. The greatest literary work of the South India Siddhas, the *Tirumandiram*, advocates a path of purification, by which the fire of inner aspiration for the Lord consumed everything else.

As a progressive path, one gradually becomes closer to the Lord, through service, becoming His "servant," then, through devotional activities, becoming His "friend," through Yoga, acquiring His qualities, and finally, through wisdom, becoming One with the Lord.

7. The teaching not the teacher is what is important: Jesus repeatedly emphasized that "the Kingdom of Heaven is within you." (Matthew 19.24, Mark 4.30 and Thomas 20.2-4) The theme of Jesus' teachings in the Synoptic Gospels as well as the Gospel of St Thomas is "the Kingdom of Heaven." But in the epistles of Paul, as well as the Gospel of John, which is considered by the vast majority of reputable scholars to contain only interpolations (statements put into the mouth of Jesus by unknown sources) the theme of his teachings is Jesus himself - his mission and his person. The Siddhas repeatedly taught that the Lord was to be found within oneself, as Absolute Being, Consciousness and Bliss; that this state could only be realized through the cultivation of samadhi, the breathless state of communion with God, and that the Lord was, unlike our soul, unaffected by desires and karma. The Siddhas in most cases

never spoke of their person. Being one with everything, there remained no more inclination to be special. They taught how to realize the Lord through the practice of Kundalini Yoga, the cultivation of wisdom and various spiritual disciplines to purify oneself of the egoistic perspective.

8. Transformation of the physical body into a liberated body of light: Jesus used the metaphor of Light to represent consciousness and his true identity: "I am the Light." (John 8.12) He also reportedly walked on water (Mark 6.45-52), rose from the dead, appeared to many persons for forty days thereafter, and ascended bodily into heaven. The Siddhas taught that we are Absolute Being, Consciousness and Bliss: *sat chit ananda*. The ultimate stage of spiritual development for the Siddhas was the attainment of the body of light, *divya deha,* or *cinmaya*. It is a "body" of infinite space (*vettaveli)*, a vast expanse without any determination. At this stage the "body" glows with the fire of immortality, and one is no longer subject to the forces of disease and death. It is called "the body of light." As Tirumular says figuratively, even the "hairs" of this transmuted body will shine. When a Siddha attains body of light, he attains Sivahood, Godhood. In Siddha mysticism the liberation of the soul is not conceived as being outside the physical body; rather the concept is of liberation within the span of life (*jiva mukti*).

The Siddhas taught and demonstrated that one may overcome death by developing through complete surrender to the Lord, a divine body, and consequently remain indefinitely in the world. If one eventually leaves it, it is because one is called by the Lord to leave, and not because the physical body has become diseased or has died.

9. Ascension of the physical body: The Acts of the Apostles, verse 1.9 reports that Jesus ascended bodily into heaven forty days after he rose from the dead. During these 40 days, He appeared to his disciples and performed many miracles. In John 20.26-29, "doubting Thomas" verified Jesus' corporeal nature by touching His hands. The body of Jesus was not buried. Although rare in the Jewish tradition, ascent into heaven is recorded in the case of Enoch (Genesis 5.24) and the prophet Elijah (2 Kings 2.11) as well as in non-canonical writings of Abraham, Moses, Isaiah and Ezra.[13]

★The south Indian Saivite literature reports cases of many of its greatest saints ascending into heaven, including Manicka Vachagar (705-807 C.E.) Thirugnana Sambanthar, Muruga Nayanar, Anaaya Nayanar, Amarneethi Nayana, Kotpuli Nayanar, and later the great poetess Andal, and the great *Acharyas* (ones who teach by example) Sankara, Ramunuja, and Madhva, who all disappeared miraculously during the 9th to 11th centuries C.E. In the 19th century, the famed *Siddha* Ramalinga Swamigal recorded in detail how he had transformed his body into a divine body of light. In 1874, he disappeared in a flash of violet light. In 2003, he is reported to have reappeared briefly to a group of French scientists who visited his home in Mettukupam, Tamil Nadu.

The Siddhas sing repeatedly of how their physical bodies became transformed and immortal as a result of their complete surrender to the Lord. The Siddha Thirumoolar, the author of the *Tirumandiram* proclaimed that he lived for aeons in a divinely transformed body:

"I lived in this body for numberless *crores* of years.

I lived in a world where there is neither day nor night.

I lived under the feet of the Lord." (*Tirumandiram* verse 74)

"I have realized the blissful Grace Shakti (spiritual energy) of pure Shakti (force of God) manifest in the very flesh of body. I have realized the Master of Knowledge in unity who having become myself becomes Himself (that is, I become Himself) who is the origin of gods, and who is the excellent Light of Vastness." (*Tirumandiram* verse 2324)

"In unity I lived many aeons of life by becoming one, in my inner consciousness, with the state of the Divine, with the Supramental Heaven, and with the Consciousness Itself." (*Tirumandiram* verse 2953)[14]

★What happened to Jesus at the end of his life is also a part of his teaching. According to the Siddhas, after death, one may go to one of many heavens or lower astral planes where one may suffer. But eventually, in order to fulfill one's latent desires, the soul is drawn back into reincarnation. However, one may be liberated from this cycle of reincarnation by becoming a liberated soul (*jivan mukta*). A truly liberated soul, they taught, is however, "the man liberated while living".[15]

In *Tirumandiram* we find a description of the characteristics of a *jivan mukta*. In Siddha philosophy there is no liberation at the time of leaving one's body (*videha-mukti*), but only liberation while living, (*jivan mukti*) or attaining immortality, while living by transforming the physical body into a divine body, a *divya deha;* for post-mortem liberation, *videha mukti* can only be at best, a hypothesis. No one can confirm it after one has died. In Siddha philosophy a *jivan mukta* does not die to attain liberation, but is transformed into the very mode of liberation, viz., the *divya deha*. When the liberated soul takes on the divine body, he becomes one with Eternity, supremely free. The "either-or" category of logic regarding his existence or non-existence does not arise in the case of a Siddha who has attained such a divine body. They have gone beyond "I am the body" perspective. A *jivan mukta,* liberated soul, does not possess a personal consciousness, but a witnessing consciousness. Even though he acts in the world, he does not have the sense of "I act." He sees all the usual things in a miraculous new light as he has entered into the heart of reality. There are outstanding examples liberated souls who attained divine bodies before disappearing from the world: Saint Nandanar, Saint Manikkavasagar, Sri Andal (merging with the Lord at Srirangam), Sri Caitanya, the Siddha Boganathar, and Ramalinga Swamigal. Sri Krisna transformed his material body into such a divine body when he desired to leave the world. He, in concentration, executed a Yoga process termed the process of radiating inner fire (a*gneyi-yoga-dharma*), by which he reduced his body to a subtler form, and with that body he left the world. This is mentioned in the "*Bhagavata.*"[16]

10. Opposition and persecution by religious authorities: Jesus was opposed to and crucified by those who ruled the temple founded by David in Jerusalem: the priests and Pharisees. They saw him as a threat to their privileged position. Jesus sought to liberate the Jews not from the Romans, but from their spiritual ignorance and fear of God. He taught them through his parables, and initiated chosen disciples into how to know God by turning within, in esoteric practices. The Siddhas have been opposed

to this day by the vested interests of Hinduism, the Brahmins, who control the temples and serve as intermediaries between the common person and the "gods" of the Hindu pantheon. The Siddhas were condemned and ridiculed by many of the Brahmins, who feared their popular appeal among the masses. The Siddhas and other yogic adepts initiate only the most qualified students into the esoteric practices of Kundalini Yoga and meditation.

11. Inner spiritual experience over scriptural authority: Jesus emphasized love and the inner experience or communion with God, rather than the law of the Old Testament. The Siddhas rejected the *Vedic* scripture's emphasis on external fire sacrifice and ritual. They rejected scripture as their ultimate authority, in place of personal mystical experience. They emphasized the inner path to the Lord through Kundalini Yoga. Both Jesus and the Siddhas taught from an expanded state of consciousness, and sought to share this state with others. Knowing that it could not communicated merely by words, spoken or written, they sought to change the perspective of their listeners, by using words and the teachings of scripture to first prepare the devotees, and then initiating the most worthy and sincere into spiritual disciplines which would give them the experience of God. God could not be known, much less captured in theological distinctions or external ritual. So, the Old Testament was not rejected by Jesus. Instead, he tried to help his listeners to go beyond the letter of the Jewish laws and commandments to its spirit. He tried to show them how to enter "the Kingdom of Heaven" by purifying themselves of all egoistic tendencies, thereby permitting one to stand in the heart of one's own highest Self. Siddha Patanjali tells us: "The Lord (*ishvara*) is the special Self, untouched by any afflictions, actions, fruits of actions (karma) or by any inner impressions of desires."[17] Therefore, if we want to know the Lord, we can do so by realizing our true Self, behind the mask of the body-mind-personality, as pure consciousness. Realizing the Self, the consciousness gradually expands and realizes the Lord as Absolute Being, Consciousness and Bliss.

12. Miracles and powers: Jesus performed many miracles as a result of his powers or siddhis. There are seven miracles in John 1-11: Water

into Wine, the Distant Boy Cured, Sickness and Sin, the Bread and the Fish, Walking on Water, the Blind Man Healed, and the Dead Man Raised. John Dominic Crossan has postulated the existence of a common source that lies behind the following miracles described in Mark and John:

Sickness and Sin	Mark 2.1-12	John 5. 1-18
Bread and Fish	Mark 6.33-44	John 6.1-15
Walking on water	Mark 6.45-52	John 6.16-21
Blind Man Healed	Mark 8.22-26	John 9.1-7
Dead Man Raised	Secret Mark 1v20-2r11a	John 11.1-57

18

Stories of Jesus curing a paralytic are found in all four narrative Gospels. That of John differs substantially from the others, yet the stories have enough in common to suggest that they stem ultimately from a common oral tradition. Scholars have generally concluded that the first miracle listed above did not include Jesus giving authority to forgive sins to his disciples.

As described in the introduction of this chapter, the Siddhas had many *siddhis* (powers) which permitted them to perform similar miracles. According to the Tamil Lexicon, *siddhi* means "realization," "success," "attainment," "final liberation." It is "attainment," or "accomplishment" connected with the super-physical worlds. In the holy hymns of south Indian Saivism, known as the *Tevaram,* the term *siddhi* means "success" in attaining God. The third chapter of the *Yoga-sutras* of Patanjali not only records sixty-eight such powers, but describes how they may be developed through a combination of cognitive absorption and concentrating on that which is desired. The *Autobiography of a Yogi*, by Paramahansa Yogananda, includes many accounts of such Yogic miracles with explanations for how they are performed according to Yogic science. Yogananda reported that his *Guru*, Sri Yukteswar, came in a transformed physical body and visited him, even though he had witnessed his burial. When

Yogananda dramatically left his from his body in 1952, in front of a crowd which included the Lieutenant Governor of California and the Ambassador of India, the Los Angeles Chief Medical Officer reported that there were no signs of physical deterioration even twenty-one days later, just before his body was put into a crypt.[19] This created a sensation in America, and was reported in Time Magazine in March, 1952.

Traditionally, *siddhis* are eight in number known as *asta siddhi*. *Asta siddhi* is of three types: two *siddhis* of knowledge (*garima* and *prakamya*), three *siddhis* of power (*isitva, vasitva* and *kamavasayitva*) and three *siddhis* of the body (*anima, mahima* and *laghima*). *Garima* is the ability to reach everywhere. *Prakayama* is freedom of will or the ability to overcome natural obstacles. *Isitva* is the ability to create or to control. *Vasitva* is the power to dominate the entire creation. *Kamavasayitva* is the ability to attain everything desired or to attain the state of desirelessness. *Anima* is the ability to become as minute as an atom. *Mahima* is the ability to expand indefinitely. *Laghima* is the power of levitation.[20]

13. Penance, self purification and the acquisition of miraculous powers: Jesus spent forty days in the wilderness in meditation and prayer, and as a result acquired great powers. The Siddhas performed similar penance (*tapas*) with resulting powers or *siddhis*. *Tapas* means "intense practice" or "austerity" and literally translates as "straightening by fire," derived from the word *tap* (to make hot). It refers to any intense or prolonged practice for Self-realization, which involves overcoming the natural tendencies of the body, emotions and mind. Because of the resistance of the body, emotions or mind, heat or pain may develop as a byproduct, but this is never the objective. Jesus reportedly was challenged by many temptations during his period of penance in the desert. (Luke 4.1-14, Mark 1.12-13, Matthew 4:1-11)

We may be learned in the sacred texts and have performed so many devotional acts, but if we have not performed *tapas*, or austerities, the senses, the mind and emotions will ultimately overwhelm our consciousness. *Tapas* is voluntary self-challenge or self-limitation - any practice that pushes the mind against its own limits is *tapas*, as when one voluntarily denies oneself of a particular desire. The postponement and eventual renunciation of the desire generates great psychic energy, which helps one to experience the inner delight behind the surface impulses of the body-mind. The key ingredient is endurance. A *tapasvin* or yogin challenges his body and mind and applies great willpower to whatever practice he vows to undertake, beginning with a vow, for example, to fast for so many hours, or to sit in meditation for a set period, or to observe silence, avoid certain activities, etc.

According to the *Bhagavad Gita* (17.14-16), there are three types of *tapas*: for body, for speech and for mind. Are they not also qualities seen in Jesus?

- Body: purity, rectitude, chastity, non-harming, making offerings to higher beings.

- Speech: speaking only kind, truthful, and beneficial words that give no offense, self observation, regular study of sacred texts, and silence.

- Mind: serenity, gentleness, silence, self-restraint, pure emotions, control of the sensual desire tendencies through the eyes, palate, hearing, nostril and skin.

By *tapas*, impurities which limit the physical, vital and mental bodies are gradually eliminated. As a result, the five subtle senses (corresponding to the physical senses) such as clairvoyance, clairaudience etc, all develop and the body becomes invulnerable, graceful and beautiful. In the *Tirumandiram* there are more than 100 different references to the perfection of the body and the senses.

Patanjali tells us in *Yoga-sutra* III.4 that *siddhis* are the result of a state of communion, with the Lord, which combines concentration, meditation and cognitive absorption (*samadhi*). Other causes he adds in IV.2 are a specific birth, herbs, mantras, and *tapas*, that is, intense practice of Yoga.

14. Public display of powers: Jesus often asked those who witnessed his display of miraculous powers, particularly, healing, not to tell anyone of what they had seen. Why? According to Patanjali, *siddhis* are marvellous accomplishments from the worldly perspective of waking consciousness, but making them one's goal creates an obstacle to the perfection of the state of s*amadhi*. (*Yoga-sutra* II.37) Like anything, they can become an object of desire, both for the possessor and those who witness them. So instead of sticking to the spiritual task of God realization, one can become diverted. There is, however, nothing intrinsically wrong in their exhibition. They are signposts along the way, for both the exhibitor and the witness. As the Siddha Pambatti says "those who have attained self realization will not exhibit it and those who have not attained self realization are those who exhibit it." Dr. Ganapathy has observed: "But to the true Siddha, who is a genuine Kundalini Yogin, these *siddhis* are of immense value, for they indicate that he is in the process of deconditioning himself from the laws of nature and from karmic determinism forever, and breaking down the structures of the profane sensibility. *Siddhi* expresses the quality of mystic experience attained by the Siddha. The real *siddhi* consists in inner conversion, an inner world of oneness, an entering into the stream of liberation. What is prohibited is not the attainment of the *siddhis* but their exhibition to others."[21]

15. Social concern and showing the spiritual path to others: Both the Siddhas and Jesus exhibited great social concern. Jesus left John the Baptist, rejecting asceticism and his belief that the end of the world was at hand; he returned to the urban areas and consorted with tax collectors and other disreputable types. He healed sick, fed the poor, and taught his listeners how they could enter the Kingdom of Heaven by purifying themselves, for example, by giving their wealth away. He encouraged counter-cultural movements against established tradition. Through his parables and teachings he gave his listeners a new, profound perspective of themselves, "the Kingdom of God," and a new social order loving everyone. The *Siddhas* sought to show the path to the Lord to everyone, by teaching what one must do to realize *samadhi*, especially through Kundalini Yoga and hygienic living standards, and medicine, and what one must avoid.

The concept, prevalent in both in the Buddhist bodhisattva vow and Tamil Siddha *arrupadai,* of showing the path to one and all irrespective of caste, creed, sex, religion, or nationality has acquired a profound social and philosophical meaning for the Siddha*s*. It is a concept emphasizing the vow of helping humanity by one's own enlightenment. Their songs and poems are indicators of the path of self-realization for the seeker of truth. The Siddhas wanted everyone to enjoy what they themselves enjoyed. They had a loving desire to secure the welfare, happiness, and solidarity of all beings. Showing others the path to spirituality is the highest altruistic action. They sincerely felt that genuine freedom is not in isolation. This is an important distinction, for most yogis in the East aspire for individual liberation *(moksha)*, to get themselves off of the karmic wheel of birth and death, the endless lifetimes, experiencing the world of sorrow. These Siddhas, on the other hand, like Jesus, aspired to show everyone the path of liberation from the endless sorrows of the world. Their aspiration was for the many to attain a one eternal, all-relating, all uniting self knowledge, i.e., a kingdom of heaven on earth. Sri Aurobindo, one of the greatest Siddhas and sages of modern times referred to this process as the "supramental evolution."

Mantras (spiritually potent sound syllable) were traditionally given only privately and only to the most deserving souls. Ramanuja, the eleventh century Indian philosopher was given initiation into a secret and powerful mantra. It was reported that he was so moved by what he had received through the mantra that he immediately went to the top of the temple tower at Srirangam, in Tamil Nadu, India, and chanted aloud the mantra so that all could hear it. In response to what he had done, the Brahmin priests threatened Ramanuja with a curse, to send his soul to hell. In reply he said that even if only one listener could receive the blessing of this mantra, he would gladly endure hell. Such is the resolve of the Siddhas.

A most powerful mantra of the Siddhas is *"sivayanama."* It is not merely a philosophical concept or mystical instrument, but a social concept too. *Nama* means sacrifice (*tyaga*), and *siva* means bliss (*ananda*). *Aya* means outcome or result. The *mantra sivayanama* thus means "the result of sacrifice is bliss.". To the Siddhas the highest form of service is the sacrifice one makes to attain Self-realization, for the whole world is sublimely benefited by it. We are all intimately connected through our thoughts and level of consciousness, not merely by words and deeds. And in sacrificing the worldly entanglements of the ego, and practicing austerities, one feels bliss, which is transmitted to all. The mystic experience of the Siddhas has given a new meaning to social service.

The *arrupadai* concept includes what one shall not do in order to achieve realization, such as taking half measures like casteism, rituals, temple worship, etc. because according to the Siddhas, much of our delusion is caused by the institutions associated with such systems. The positive aspect includes the method of Kundalini Yoga, ethical precepts, their system of medicine and their simple vernacular language conveying their teachings. In short, rather than trying to renounce the world, the Siddhas dedicated themselves to its upliftment, while enjoying perfect freedom. It represents a new paradigm for humanism on a world scale, one that is informed not by social theorists, but by divinely inspired Siddhas, or perfected mystics.[22]

The practice of an integral Yoga, as conceived by the Siddhas, has social consequences. Our thoughts, words and actions affect not only ourselves, but everyone we meet in society: friends, strangers, family members, co-workers, even people at a distance. Patanjali and the Siddhas recognized this in emphasizing social restraints (*yamas*) and observances (*niyamas*) as the foundation of ones' practice. The restraints of Yoga are: non-violence, truthfulness, non-stealing, chastity and greedlessness. The observances of Yoga are: purity, contentment, accepting but not causing pain, self-study and surrender to the Lord. Do these not reflect the same qualities and aspirations taught by Jesus?

1. *Ahimsa* (non-violence): *Himsa* means harming so *ahimsa* means non-harming. This includes avoidance of causing harm to others by thoughts, words and actions. As yogis, our thoughts and words are much more powerful than those of others, whose energies are generally dispersed. So, we should avoid thinking ill of others, or making judgments about them, as this will only reinforce whatever negative quality they have, and cause us to indulge it in ourselves. Speak, only after reflection, what is helpful and uplifting.

Right action will then follow right thought and speech. *Ahimsa* may include protecting others from harm.

2. *Satya* (truthfulness): Express only what is true, and avoid lying, exaggeration, deceit, hypocrisy and pretension - truth in advertising. Otherwise we deceive ourselves, postpone the working out of existing *karma*, and create or reinforce new *karmic* consequences. By leaving aside all fiction, all imaginary or unreal things, in mind, speech and action, one quickly discovers the truth. To speak only what is true is very revealing. Use words to bless others. Speak, after reflection, what comes from your heart or higher self. This brings clarity to our minds and relationships.

3. *Asteya* (non-stealing): This includes avoiding taking something that does not belong to oneself. Stealing engulfs our consciousness with darkness, wherein we fail to see our essential unity. It closes our heart, strengthens egoistic tendencies, and drives us away from the path of Self-realization.

4. *Brahmacharya* (chastity): This involves sexual abstinence in the physical, emotional and vital, as well as mental, planes. Its cultivation facilitates letting go of what is usually a great source of distraction and suffering for most persons, and consequently aids the process of Self-realization. Even if one lives in a committed relationship with a partner, if one can cultivate moderation and awareness in one's sexual relations, most distraction and dispersion can be avoided. One loves the other as one's Self. One must be careful to avoid suppression and to develop antipathy towards others, or feelings of guilt, shame or frustration with regards to sexual impulses. Reflect deeply on the nature of sexuality and take a holistic approach in using it.

5. *Aparigrahah* (greedlessness): This includes not fantasizing over material possessions, nor coveting things belonging to others. Often people fantasize about how much happier their life would be if they won the lottery, made a big profit in the stock market, or

married a rich person. Such fantasies simply distract one from the inner source of joy.[23]

The *niyamas* or "observances of Classical Yoga" are described by Patanjali in *Yoga-Sutra* II.32 as:

1. *Sauca* (purity): involves body, mind and speech. Patanjali tells us that through it one develops detachment towards one's own body, "sattva" or beingness, the basis for illumination, as well as joy, concentration, and mastery over the senses. Jesus tells us "blessed are the pure in heart for they shall see God." (Matthew 5:8)

2. *Santosha* (contentment): an inner poise wherein there is neither liking nor disliking. Patanali tells us that it brings supreme joy.

3. *Tapas* (accepting but not causing pain): reminds us of the saying of Jesus to "turn the other cheek," when one harms you. Patanjali tells us that through it, perfection is attained.

4. *Svadhyaya* (self study): involves the study of the sacred literature, which serves as a mirror for our higher Self, or soul, as well remembering to let go of what one is not, the reactions of the mind, emotions and body. Through it, Patanjali tells us, one is able to commune with the Lord. Jesus' teachings also referred to the sacred scriptures, as a tool for remembering who we truly are, and our relationship with the Lord.

5. *Ishvara-pranidhana* (surrender to the Lord): through it Patanjali assures us, one attains *samadhi* or cognitive absorption, referred to by Jesus as "the Kingdom of Heaven." This reminds us of the biblical admonition to love the Lord with all of your heart, all your mind, and in everything you do. Jesus constantly taught his listeners how to love God.

Was Jesus a Guru?

Jesus accepted Mary Magdalene as a disciple when he allowed her to wash and anoint his feet. He initiated his most worthy disciples into esoteric teachings enabling them to realize the Supreme Being, beyond the creator god. The Siddhas showed their surrender to their Gurus by washing or touching their feet. They initiated their disciples into advanced techniques of Yoga to expand their consciousness and bring about Self-realization. The Gnostic Gospel of Thomas, the Gospel of Mary, and the recently discovered Gospel of Judas reveal how Jesus initiated his most advanced disciples into secret "knowledge" or gnosis.

Here are excerpts from the Gospel of Judas, written around 140 A. D:

"During the *eucharist* meal, three days before the Passover, Jesus puts His twelve disciples to a test, challenging anyone of them to stand before Him and tell Him who He is. Only Judas dares to, and said: 'I know who you are and where you have come from. You are from the immortal realm of Barbelo. I am not worthy to utter the name of the one who has sent you.' Knowing that Judas was reflecting upon something that was exalted, Jesus said to him, 'Step away from the others and I shall tell you the mysteries of the kingdom. It is possible for you to reach it, but you will grieve a great deal. For someone else will replace you, in order that the twelve disciples may again come to completion with their god.'"[24]

"Later Jesus took Judas aside. Jesus said, "Come, that I may teach you about secrets no person has ever seen. For there exists a great and boundless realm, whose extent no generation of angels has seen, in which there is a great invisible Spirit." And a luminous cloud appeared there."[25]

Initiation into Yoga is referred to as *diksa,* and it is given by the initiator, the Guru, in the Siddha tradition. To understand Jesus, one has to understand the meaning of the Sanskrit word *Guru.* The Sanskrit term *Guru* is derived from two roots: *gu* (darkness) and *ru* (light). A Guru removes the darkness of ignorance or non-truth and leads his pupil towards enlightenment and truth. It is a principle of nature by which one realizes the truth of things. It may express itself through any situation or thing that creates wisdom. In truth, wisdom is the Guru. One may experience the Guru as "pure love," while looking in your baby's eyes; or while absorbed in the absolute beauty of a sunrise or sunset over the ocean, or while reading scripture, or through the eyes or words of a saint. A surge of Pure Love, Pure Awareness, Absolute Beauty, Compassion, Absolute Peace, Truth, these are experiences of the guru principle at work.

When this kind of awareness expresses consistently through an individual human being, that person may become known as a Guru, but it is what comes through that person which has the power to transform others. A true Guru does not identify himself or herself with the body-mind-personality, and is, like Jesus, humbly a servant of the Lord. Knowing that they have transcended both name and form. Becoming one with everything, one is identified with All. When all conditioning of the ego is gone, as in the case of the greatest of Siddhas, there is nothing to misinterpret the truth. Truth flows through these beings, pure and unadulterated, straight from God. Rarest on earth are such individuals.

Most devotees and even disciples do not realize the Truth of these individuals on earth, and the person of their teacher remains an enigma. So they make the mistake of worshipping the teacher rather than the teachings. Such was the case, for example, of Gautama Buddha, who sought to replace overemphasis on worship in Hinduism with wisdom teachings about suffering and desire, and subsequently became an object of worship. It is for this reason that the greatest of wisdom teachers, the highest Gurus, withdraw after awhile from public access, and keep their own "story" obscure. It is imbibing and living the wisdom of the teachings, not worshipping the teacher which is important for the world.

The Guru is a spiritual preceptor who initiates his disciples onto the spiritual path and guides them towards liberation. The Guru is one who has realized his identity with That, the absolute source of everything, and assumes the responsibility of guiding others to that realization. As such, God manifests in the form of the Guru. The Grace of God is the Guru.

The Guru is the principle by which Nature creates, sustains and destroys all life in both our inner and outer universes, in whatever way is necessary for us to pass from ignorance to wisdom, from egoism to Self-realization. It has existed since before the universe was created, and so transcends time and space. The Guru principle exists within everyone as the inner Self, so when we honor the outer Guru, we also honor our own Self.

Mircea Eliade characterises Yoga as "initiatory structure." A better translation of *diksa* is "empowerment," because in it the teacher carries the pupil in himself, like a mother who carries the embryo in her womb and "empowers" the disciple with all his *jnana* (wisdom) energy. The term *diksa* is a compound of two ideas, *diyate* and *ksiyate* – giving and weakening. One gives or imparts knowledge, and weakens or destroys lower impulses and desires, the obstacles or fetters to enlightenment and liberation. Initiation is a spiritual rebirth, which begins a long process of transformation. In the *Siddha* tradition initiation involves training in Kundalini Yoga, which includes in particular breathing exercises performed while visualizing the circulation of energy through the most important subtle channels, or *nadis,* the *ida, pingala, sushumna*, located in the spine of the physical body. It also involves initiation into mantras for *chakras*, the seven psycho-energetic centers, and specialized meditation techniques and postures designed to awaken a spark of potential spiritual energy, known as the *kundalini,* which lies coiled and dormant at the base of the spine. The Guru is considered to be the primary threshold in the ascent of the staircase to liberation.

The Siddhas worshiped their Gurus. This fact distinguishes them and other followers of the *Tantra* faith from the followers of the *Vedic* faith who are called *devabhaju* or the worshippers of the demigods or *devas.* One of the distinguishing features of the Siddhas was that nowhere in their literary works do they sing the praise of any local gods or deities. The Guru arises essentially as a vastness of space (*vettaveli*), freedom or wisdom in which the disciple loses himself. Sometimes the lineage of the previous Gurus may itself stand for the Guru: that is, the Guru need not necessarily be a living human being. The Guru not only teaches students how to meditate, to be aware, but continues to encourage them throughout the process of practicing, realizing, purifying, until one attains Self-realization. The Guru, according to the *Siddha* tradition, is not a repository of knowledge, a mere expert; he is an authority who has experienced the truth and attained Self-realization, and is then called to guide others towards Self-realization.

Jesus was not merely a teacher or rabbi to his disciples, but a God-man, who remained an enigma to all of his direct disciples. Jesus was initiated by John the Baptist at the time of his baptism in the Jordan River. He was given a powerful spiritual experience as a result of John's empowerment. Jesus in turn exhibited the powers and functions of a Guru in the Indian tradition of the Yoga Siddhas.

The disciples of Jesus struggled to comprehend his teachings, his parables, and referred to him variously as a prophet, or the messiah, foretold in the Old Testament, the anointed one who would deliver them from the yoke of Roman tyranny. His public ministry lasted less than two years. They therefore had very little time to mature and grasp who he was before He was gone. Their confusion and debate over who Jesus was lead to the formation of a multiplicity of sects in early Christianity, based upon various answers to the questions of "Who was Jesus?" Was He God? Was he a man? Was he both God and man? The debate raged until the third century A.D., when the Church, in alliance with the Roman emperor, began to define its dogma and to declare those who did not adhere to its dogma as heretics. Sometimes, a physical Guru merges with the Absolute Being Consciousness and Bliss, leaving the physical plane, yet, remains able and willing to help true aspirants. The Guru in subtle form remains, as the grace-bestowing power of God. Guru, God, Self, all pervading consciousness, *shakti* - are all one. God, Guru, Self, All Pervading Consciousness, Jesus-are all one.

Jesus clearly exhibited all of the above characteristics of a Guru. The fact that the term *guru* has become anathema for orthodox Western Christians is in itself indicative of the effect that such God-men have upon those who are bound by religious convention. How can a human being also be God? This paradox caused over three hundred years of debate in early Christianity, and still today provokes a hue and cry of "sacrilege" and "charlatan" from modern day Pharisees.

The term "*Guru*" has often become a term of disrespect largely because the leaders of conventional and orthodox religions as well as cynics and other professional doubters in the media feel threatened by anyone who claims to have special knowledge of Truth. While this is especially so in the West, where knowledge is power, it is still the case in all cultures where organized religion's leaders leave little room for the unorthodox, the radicals and the mystics. If Jesus was to return today, he would undoubtedly be deemed as another "Guru" by the above cited modern day Pharisees. He would probably also aim at them parables drawn from contemporary culture and sage retorts. He would attract some and repel others. He might even be investigated by the security services and tax authorities, in some countries. He would undoubtedly be ridiculed and even persecuted by the orthodox religious.

●Orthodox Christianity systematically eradicated Gnostics and their writings - those who, like Jesus, claimed to have found a special inner knowledge. While orthodox Christianity tolerated its mystics, as long as they remained quiet, in their monasteries, it has continued to replace the message of Jesus, that "the Kingdom of Heaven is within you," with the message of Paul and John: that by believing in the Lord Jesus Christ, your sins are forgiven and you are saved from eternal damnation. Until and unless the authentic teachings of Jesus are restored to their rightful place, many sincere seekers of God and truth will continue to look to "Gurus" outside of Christianity for the special inner knowledge which leads to the Kingdom of Heaven. Ultimately the disciple, yogi or Christian, must one day go beyond the external Guru and discover the inner Guru, which is the principle that reveals the wisdom from within.

Devotees Versus Disciples

Jesus had only a handful of disciples, including the twelve Apostles and Mary Magdalene. Many others, however, heard his message, took it to heart, and revered him. These were his devotees. A disciple is one who goes further however, and dedicates himself or herself to the prescribed discipline. While Jesus did not ask his listeners to abandon the Jewish law or practices, he did insist on applying oneself wholeheartedly to its underlying spirit. For those who understood this, he offered secret teachings, or initiations, during which they were empowered to realize this spiritual dimension of reality. Jesus, like the Yoga Siddhas, reserved the sharing of his most sublime spiritual truths for disciples in personal sessions of initiation. During these, a true communion occurs between the Guru and the disciple. The spirit has no form, so any attempt to reduce these experiences into creeds or symbols only serves to distract from the essence of the teaching. By applying oneself to the prescribed spiritual disciplines, however, disciples can repeatedly renew their communion with spiritual truth, "beyond names and forms." This truth remains an enigma for the uninitiated.

Are There Any Differences Between Jesus and the Yoga Siddhas?

These are relatively minor, as we will see. While we have been comparing the *teachings* of Jesus and Siddhas, it is also instructive to compare their *lives*, given that one's life is the best form that a teaching can possibly take.

- Jesus did not record in writing any of his teachings. He wrote no Gospel. Instead, he preached. The *Siddhas* recorded their teachings often in the form of poems or stories, which could be easily memorized by the common people, and wrote them in palm leaf manuscripts.

- Jesus, as far as we know, did not travel outside the region of modern-day Israel. The *Siddhas* traveled not only all over India, by their own accounts, traveled also to China, Southeast Asia, Arabia, and southern Europe.

- Jesus, as far as we know, did not have a Guru, unless one considers John the Baptist to have been so. He did not attribute his wisdom to anyone else, unless one considers the Old Testament prophets to have been such a source. John the Baptist baptized Jesus, initiating him into the experience of divine communion, when the Holy Spirit descended upon him in the form of a dove.

- The Siddhas revered their Gurus as the source of their wisdom. We know that the Siddhas developed and transmitted the methods of Yoga, especially Kundalini Yoga and meditation, to their disciples. We do not know what methods or *gnosis* Jesus may have imparted to his most worthy disciples during secret initiations.

- Jesus lived only thirty three years. His short ministry was cut short with his crucifixion on the cross. His ministry lasted only about one year. He left his disciples in disarray and confused, ill prepared to teach as He taught. The Siddhas, by their own accounts, are reported to have lived for hundreds of years. Jesus lived during the first century; scholars place the Siddha Patanjali somewhere around 200 B.C.; Siddha Agastyar was spoken of in the RigVeda, written around 1500 B.C. after having been transmitted orally for many thousands of years. The Upanishads of the Rishis were written between 1000 B.C. and 500 C.E. Siddha Thirumular completed writing the *Thirumandiram* in the fourth century C.E. The *Siddha* Goraknath lived around the eleventh century C.E.

- Jesus spoke Aramaic, and was raised as a Jew. He observed the Jewish Laws, but not always, as he often criticized them or recommended that their underlying purpose be realized: respecting the Law's spirit if not its letter. The Siddhas were raised in traditions which are part of the federation of faiths known today as Hinduism, or *sanatana dharma* (eternal righteous way). Like Jesus, however, they held to experience as the ultimate source of authority.

- Jesus never married, as far as we know. He was an itinerant teacher of wisdom. The *Siddhas* were often householders, at least for some period of their lives. They made their contributions to the world in a variety of professions, medicine, literature, and various sciences.

- Jesus was crucified, rose from the dead, and eventually ascended into heaven, according to the Gospel writers. The Siddhas, though often censured by the orthodox, were not persecuted, lived long lives, and in many cases disappeared or "ascended" miraculously.

Was Jesus a Yoga Siddha?

While there is no conclusive evidence that Jesus ever visited India, the traditional homeland of Yoga, or learned anything termed "Yoga," the many similarities, described above, between Jesus and the Siddhas, leaves little doubt that Jesus exemplified almost all of the resultant qualities of one who has become a "perfected" human being, a Siddha. He was much more than a saint and a sage, and still much more than a prophet or teacher of wisdom. His miracles and powers, his absence of egoism, and manner of teaching all suggest one who has reached the pinnacle of perfection, *siddhi*. The fact that few can even begin to grasp how such a perfection could be accomplished is one of the resulting mysteries of his missing years, prior to his public ministry. This gap in our knowledge of his formative years also suggests why so many have projected upon Jesus the role of their Savior, though, as we will see in subsequent chapters, He never claimed in any authenticated saying, to be anyone's Savior. The mystery of his missing years also suggests that he purposefully never revealed where these years were spent.

One need not go to another land, another culture, to find the truth, to find the Kingdom of Heaven. The short cut to the Kingdom of Heaven, Jesus taught, was within oneself. Ironically, this teaching, his most profound message for the world was lost in the Christian doctrine that rose up around his personage. What is important to note is that this same message comes from the teachings of the Siddhas and all other adepts of wisdom traditions around the world. What is important to note is that the Siddhas and other adepts indicate similar spiritual disciplines to anyone aspiring to that Kingdom of Heaven on earth.

CHAPTER 3

Gospel of Thomas: A Gnostic Text?

The Gospel of Thomas is widely considered by scholars to contain many of the original sayings of Jesus. It was discovered in 1945 among the Gnostic texts at Nag Hammadi in Upper Egypt. Consisting of one hundred and fourteen sayings, and unlike the other Gospels whose authors are unknown, according to a consensus of scholars, it was recorded by, Didymos Judas Thomas, who was identified particularly within the Syrian Church as the apostle Thomas and twin brother of Jesus.[1] According to the Gnostic text, Acts of Thomas, he was also the founder of the churches in India, and was martyred near present day Chennai, south India.[2] However, according to most scholars, like the authors of the canonical gospels, the author of the Gospel of Thomas was probably not the Apostle Thomas, but someone writing in his name. Also unlike other early Christian Gospels, which typically consist of narrative accounts interpreting the life of Jesus of Nazareth and culminating in descriptions of his death, the Gospel of Thomas contains only his sayings, beginning with saying number one:

"Whoever discovers the interpretation of these sayings will not taste death."

This first saying offers the reader immortality as the prize to whomsoever can interpret these sayings correctly. The readers of the Gospel of Thomas are invited to join the quest for the meaning of life by interpreting the often cryptic and enigmatic sayings of Jesus.

The second saying warns us that the quest for realization is difficult but when completed, we will find God:

Jesus said, "Let one who seeks not stop seeking until one finds. When one finds, one will be troubled. When one is troubled, one will marvel and will rule over all."

The correct interpretation is to be gained with the aid of a special, hidden, inner knowledge. Words themselves are inadequate, but can point to truths that lie beyond the power the words have to communicate. In this quest, the seekers find themselves and God. They discover that God's kingdom is within themselves as well as spread out everywhere, and that they are "the children of the living father."

The writings of the Siddas like those of Jesus are merely "keys" to open the door to otherwise inaccessible truth and wisdom. For the most part yogic aspirants, must be initiated into the techniques of contemplation and meditation necessary to unlock the doors to the wisdom contained in the Siddhas writings. These writings point to truths that cannot be adequately expressed in words, but can be realized in higher states of consciousness during deep meditation.

We will compare several of these obscure Siddha poems with the cryptic sayings and parables of Jesus. But first, let us explore the history and significance of one of Christianity's greatest discoveries in modern times.

History and Distinctiveness of the Gospel of Thomas

The papyrus manuscript discovered in a jar in a cliff near Nag Hammadi, in the Upper Sinai desert of Egypt in 1945, was written in Coptic, and was dated to the early second century. Fragments of this Gospel were also found at Oxyrhynchus, Egypt, written in Greek, and published in 1897 and 1904. These contained many of the same verses as the Coptic edition. The one hundred and fourteen sayings in the Gospel of Thomas are presented in what appears to be more or less random order. It was composed around the end of the first century or the beginning of the second century C.E. although an earlier edition probably was composed between 50 and 60 C.E.[3]

As a collection of sayings of Jesus, the Gospel of Thomas is closer in genre to the other ancient collections of sayings, than to the New Testament Gospels. In the ancient world, going back to the third millennium B.C., Jewish, Greco-Roman and Christian collections of sayings circulated widely as wisdom literature. Proverbs, Ecclesiastes and The Wisdom of Solomon were compiled by Jewish sages in this genre of wisdom sayings. Memorable wise sayings, cynical and witty, known as *chreia* (from the Greek *chreiodes*: "useful") were created by Greek and Roman philosophers. The most well know Christian collection of sayings is what Burton Mack called "the lost Gospel" of Q, for *Quelle* (German – "source") which scholars consider to have been the primary common source, along with Mark, for many of the statements in Matthew and Luke. However, The Gospel of Thomas is completely independent from the *Q* collection of sayings.

As a Gospel of wisdom, it proclaims a distinctive message. Unlike the way in which he is portrayed in the New Testament Gospels, "Jesus in the Gospel of Thomas performs no physical miracles, reveals no fulfillment of prophecy, announces no apocalyptic kingdom about to disrupt the world order, and dies for no one's sins."[4] It is counter-cultural wisdom, and it is intended to shock its audience out of their complacent world view. It criticizes end of the world prophecies (sayings 51, 52, 113) and offers a way of salvation through communion with its sayings. It is a book of mystical wisdom, in which the world is contrasted with the kingdom of heaven, light with darkness. It echoes other mystical wisdom literature from the Gnostics, the Jewish Essenes and the Yogis of India. It contains no commentaries, unlike the canonical Gospels, whose authors cleverly interpret the sayings of Jesus for others.

The Gospel of Thomas: A Gnostic Text?

Until the discovery of the twelve codices in their original bindings at Nag Hammadi, our knowledge of the Gnostics (from the Greek *gnosis*, "knowledge"), a modern designation for a religious movement of the early centuries of the common era, was limited to the refutations of it in early Church writings. Except for a few fragments, all Gnostic writings were systematically destroyed, after being declared as heretical, or "false knowledge." A false knowledge, however, implies the existence of a true knowledge, and Clement of Alexandria in fact uses the term "Gnostic" for a Christian who has penetrated more deeply than the ordinary believer into the knowledge of the truth. (*Stromata* 7.1-2) Most of the forty works therein were Gnostic in nature.

The chief characteristics common to Gnosticism are:

- A radical cosmic dualism that rejects this world and all that belongs to it: the body is a prison from which the soul longs to escape.
- A distinction between the unknown transcendent true God and the Creator, or Demiurge, commonly identified with the God of the Hebrew Bible.
- The belief that the human race is essentially akin to the divine, being a spark of heavenly light imprisoned in a material body.
- A myth, often narrating a pre-mundane fall, to account for the present human predicament.
- The saving knowledge by which deliverance is effected and the Gnostic awakened to recognition of his or her true nature and heavenly origin.

The Nag Hammadi documents suggest that the majority of Gnostics lived ascetic lives. The classic period of Gnosticism was the second century C.E. with such figures as Basilides and Valentinus, and the latter's disciples Ptolemy and Heracleon, but this was the culmination of a long development.

Gnosticism was a religious movement in antiquity that infiltrated a number of religious traditions, including Judaism and Christianity. The British scholar E.R. Dodds characterized Gnosticism as a movement whose writings derived from mystical experience. Gershom Scholem, Professor of Jewish Mysticism at the Hebrew University in Jerusalem, agrees with Dodds that Gnosticism involves mystical speculation and practice.[5] Fundamental to the Gnostic outlook was the conviction that the world is evil. As it matured, it speculated about a variety of problems. It expressed a conviction that the world was created by an evil creator god, a fallen angel turned from the One True God. In Jewish Gnosticism, this evil creator god was named Yahweh, and he concealed the truth about Adam and Eve. The serpent was regarded as good, because he attempted to enlighten the first humans about the heavenly reality that lay beyond the evil creation of Yahweh. The serpent was therefore a savior figure. In Christian Gnosticism, Jesus Christ became this savior figure.

It is perhaps best to describe the Gospel of Thomas as reflecting a budding Gnosticism. The influence of Gnostic theology is clearly present in it. But in many ways it is not Gnostic at all. It has no doctrine of creation, no account of the fall, nothing about an evil creator God. Its saying and parables have Gnostic tendencies. The Gospel of Thomas, according to the consensus of scholars, represents an early stage in Christian Gospel writing and theologizing, quite comparable to what we find in the New Testament, especially in Paul and the Gospel of John. Its sayings indicate a Gnostic influence.

In his commentary on the Gospel of Thomas, the eminent Jewish scholar, Harold Bloom states:

"The deepest teaching of this Gnostic Jesus is never stated but always implied, implied in nearly every saying. There is light in you, and that light is no part of the created world. It is not Adamic. I know of only two convictions essential to the Gnosis: Creation and fall were part of the same event, and what is best in us was never created, so cannot fall. The American religion, Gnosis of our Evening-Land, adds a third element if our freedom is to be complete. That ultimate spark of the pre-created light must be alone, or at least alone with Jesus."[6]

These comments echo those of Indian *Samkhya*, the dualistic philosophy underlying Classical *Yoga*, wherein the Seer, *purusha* (the individual soul), is represented as the light of individualized consciousness, as distinct from the Seen, everything else, *prakriti* (Nature).[7] It also echoes Patanjali's *kaivalyam* (absolute freedom, or aloneness), the goal of Yoga:[8] There exists in most religious and many spiritual traditions, a curious opposition between "the spirit and the flesh." There is a bias against Nature, particularly against human nature. This bias has prevented many commentators and religious teachers to see the great potential for Self-realization and God-realization to transform Nature. They have for the most part concluded that the final state of realization must necessarily involve a departure from the physical plane. Certainly this was the view of the Gnostics. As we shall see, however, this view was not shared by the Yoga Siddhas. Sri Aurobindo called the ultimate state of realization, *kaivalyam* "Absolute Unity."[9] The Siddha Thirumular referred to one's true form as *svarupa*, "self-illuminating manifestness." A divorce of the spirit and the flesh may be our ordinary state, but it is not the final one, nor is it the goal. Jesus and the Siddhas show us how to marry the two.

Among the most important messages and themes, as translated by Marvin Meyers in his book, "The Gospel of Thomas":

The Kingdom of Heaven is Already Here

Saying 3:

Jesus said, "If your leaders say to you, 'Look, the kingdom is in Heaven,' then the birds of Heaven will precede you. If they say to you, 'It is in the sea,' then the fish will precede you. Rather, the kingdom is inside you and it is outside you. When you know yourselves, then you be known, and you will understand that you are children of the living father. But if you do not know yourselves, then you dwell in poverty, and you are poverty."

Saying 113:

His followers said to Him, "When will the Kingdom come?"

"It will not come by watching for it. It will not be said, 'Look, here it is,' or 'Look, there it is.' Rather, the Father's Kingdom is spread out upon the earth, and people do not see it."

Saying 51:

His followers said to Him, "When will the rest for the dead take place, and when will the new world come?"

He said to them, "What you look for has come, but you do not know it."

Jesus emerges not as a prophet using apocalyptic images to announce the end of the world and the coming of God's Kingdom, but "the good news" that this Kingdom is already a present reality. Jesus did so, while wandering from place to place, preaching with parables and clever sayings of wisdom designed to oblige his listeners to face a new and compelling vision of life.

Saying 42:

Be passerby.

To be "a passerby" is essentially a call to be detached, and to see things from a new perspective. Such detachment can take the external form of renunciation of the world, but not necessarily. What is necessary, Jesus appears to be saying, is that there must be an inner detachment if one wants to enter into the ever present "Kingdom of Heaven." Why? As Patanjali states in his *Yoga-Sutras,* until one ceases to identify with the movements of the mind, one cannot enter into the state of *samadhi*, (cognitive absorption), which Jesus referred to as "the Kingdom of Heaven."[10] In Yoga we too say, be a passerby, be as a passenger in a transit lounge merely awaiting the next event on your journey. Only in that way will one be ready to pass into the Kingdom of Heaven. The mind of man must become pure, large, tranquil, impersonal, to create a similar tranquilizing influence on the parts of our life. A mental change must lead not only into an inner status of quietude, but also an outer. To enter the Kingdom of Heaven, the mind itself must become spiritualized. To become spiritualized, the mind must become impersonal so the senses lose their hold on the world of names and forms. A conscious control over the energies of our lower nature is required. A spiritualized consciousness is only achieved when the life falls quiet, the body ceases to need and the mind ceases to identify with its emotional being and its ego's limited consciousness. The individual self of a "passerby" identifies with that, which is much greater than the mind, emotions and ego. The passerby, is the silent observer that identifies with no thing, but merely lies behind watching it All. This witnessing state of consciousness opens us into the vast space of light and knowledge. As long as one remains attached to the busyness of the world, to the business of living, one will remain blind to that, which is behind it, pure awareness. It is awareness of the witnessing state of consciousness, which Jesus wants us to acquire.

As demonstrated in the next chapter on "Early Christianity" both the Gnostic and orthodox forms of Christianity could emerge as variant interpretations of the teachings and significance of Jesus. Those attracted to solitude would note that as a prototype, Jesus was a homeless man who rejected His own family, avoided marriage and family life, a mysterious wanderer who insisted on truth at all costs, even the cost of His own life. He also demanded that others who followed him must also give up everything: family, home, children, ordinary work and wealth, to join him.[11]

In *The Historical Jesus*, John Dominic Crossan expands upon this basic assessment of Jesus: "His strategy, implicitly for himself and explicitly for his followers, was the combination of *free healing and common eating*, a religious and economic egalitarianism that negated alike and at once the hierarchical and patronal normalcies of Jewish religion and Roman power… Miracle and parable, healing and eating were calculated to force individuals into unmediated physical and spiritual contact with God and unmediated physical and spiritual contact with one another. He announced in other words, the broker less Kingdom of God."[12] The Yoga Siddhas also denounced the influence which the priests, casteism and temple worship had in the lives of the people. They taught that one could realize the Lord, as *satchidananda* (Being, Consciousness and Bliss) directly, by going inside into the state of cognitive absorption, *samadhi* without any social intermediary.

The Hidden, Gnostic Heart of the Gospel of Thomas: Jesus as Initiator of His Most Worthy Disciples into Esoteric Knowledge - Gnosis

Saying 13:

Jesus said to his followers, "Compare me to something and tell me what I am like." Simon Peter said to Him, "You are like a just messenger." Matthew said to Him, "You are like a wise philosopher." Thomas said to him, "Teacher, my mouth is utterly unable to say what you are like." Jesus said, "I am not your teacher. Because you have drunk, you have become intoxicated from the bubbling spring that I have tended." And He took him, and withdrew, and spoke three sayings to him.

When Thomas came back to his friends, they asked him, "What did Jesus say to you?" Thomas said to them, "If I tell you one of the sayings He spoke to me, you will pick up rocks and stone me, and fire will come from the rocks and consume you."

On this saying, Harold Bloom, has written:

"The living Jesus of the Gospel of Thomas speaks to all his followers, but in the crucial thirteenth saying he speaks to Thomas alone, and those secret three sayings are never revealed to us. Here we must surmise, since those three solitary sayings are the hidden heart of the Gospel of Thomas.

Thomas has earned knowledge of the sayings (or words) by denying any similitude for Jesus. His twin is not like a just messenger or prophet, nor is he like a wise philosopher, or teacher of Greek wisdom. The sayings then would turn upon the nature of Jesus: what he is. He is so much of the light as to be the light, but not the light of heaven, or of the heaven above heaven. The identification must be with the stranger or alien God, not the God of Moses and of Adam, but the man-god of the abyss, prior to creation. Yet that is only one truth out of three, though quite enough to be stoned for, and then avenged by divine fire. The second saying must be the call of that stranger God to Thomas, and third must be the response of Thomas, which is his realization that he already is in the place of rest, alone with his twin."[13]

When Thomas said to him, "Teacher, my mouth is utterly unable to say what you are like," and Jesus replied, "I am not your teacher. Because you have drunk, you have become intoxicated from the bubbling spring that I have tended," Jesus is telling Thomas that he has found himself the source of divine wisdom which will free him, just as a thirsty man finds a spring, and drinks from it. It is significant that Jesus says: "I am not your teacher." In saying this, Jesus is saying that the Lord himself is the teacher, and that Thomas has himself grasped the truth which will lead him to the Lord. Jesus attributes no special status to himself; he adopts no role. Because he knows that there is nothing which divides him from anyone or anything else. Jesus is not the teacher and he is not the teaching. The wisdom which he is sharing is. This reminds me of what happened when many persons came to the 20th century sage, Ramana Maharshi. They would ask him questions like: "Are you my guru?" He would reply with statements like: "Find out who is asking the question, and you will have your answer." The answer was not "out there." It was nothing that could be put in words. It was the realization of one's true Self, of who we were before we were born!

That there are secret, esoteric teachings revealed by Jesus to only the most advanced of his disciples is further supported by Saying 62:

Jesus said, "I disclose my mysteries to those (who are worthy) of (my) mysteries. Do not let your left hand know what your right hand is doing."

So, Jesus also acted as initiator into the mystical Gnosis, or inner knowing. Such an initiation could not have been limited to mere words, and hence they are not recordable as sayings or written teachings. The transmission of consciousness and energy by Jesus during such initiations alone could reveal to the recipient disciple the "knowledge" of one's oneness with the Supreme Being, who is beyond names and creation. This closely parallels the initiations into the esoteric methods of Yoga, given by the Yoga Siddhas to their disciples, which permit one to know the Lord as one's own highest Self.

Compare this with *Thirumandiram,* verse 2697 wherein our true identity is revealed:

> "Himself as Lord
>
> In all things, He alone is;
>
> Himself is Yourself
>
> Thus you seek Him;
>
> The very Heaven is He in this vast earth;
>
> Sweet is He;
>
> May you Him adore".

And as to the role of the Guru, (*Thirumandiram*, verse 2670):

> "Like a lustrous ray of red gem
>
> On to a green stone set
>
> Is the Holy Guru's *jnana* (wisdom) precept;
>
> That ray in the eye-brow Centre is;
>
> It is the Light within the Light Resplendent".

Mark relates that Jesus concealed his teaching from the masses, and entrusted it only to the few he considered worthy to receive it, in verses Mark 4.11, 7.17-23, 9.28-29, and 13.1-37.

Discounting the Value of Prophecy and its Fulfillment for our Freedom

Saying 52:

His followers said to Him, "Twenty-four prophets have spoken in Israel, and they all spoke of you."

He said to them, "You have disregarded the Living One who is in your presence and have spoken of the dead."

Jesus tells us it is not through prophecy that we are to find the Truth of this world, but by recognizing here and now the "Living One."

"The Living One" is not a thing, nor is it a person. It is That which exists always, throughout all the vicissitudes of life, amidst all its forms and incarnations. Light is a metaphor for it. It is the mystery of Consciousness, as distinct from body and mind. It illuminates all, yet just as we ignore the light in a room, preferring to focus on the trivial, transitory objects of this world that can be seen, or experienced through the five senses, so also, we ignore the Presence, the Truth of our true identity: *sat chit ananda* (absolute being, consciousness and bliss). It is this "Living One" which frees us from the darkness of spiritual ignorance, our confusion of being identified with a body and a mind.

Jesus does not praise the prophets. Of men, he commends only John the Baptist and his own brother, James the Just. There is no nostalgia in any of the sayings of Jesus for the virtues of the fathers of Israel. Rather, he warns us against being caught in meaningless repetition of past traditions. He has little use of institutions, titles, organizations, or positions of honor.

Who Am I?

In the Gospel of Thomas, Jesus reveals his true identity, before that of Adam, as well as our own;

Saying 77:

Jesus said, "I am the light that is over all things. I am all: From me all has come forth, and to me all has reached. Split a piece of wood; I am there. Lift up the stone, and you will find me there."

And he tells us who we truly are:

Saying 50:

Jesus said, "If they say to you, "Where have you come from?" say to them, "We have come from the Light, from the place where the Light came into being by itself, established (itself), and appeared in their image. If they say to you, "Is it you?" say, "We are its children, and we are the chosen of the living Father'" If they ask you, "What is the evidence of your Father in you?" say to them, "It is motion and rest.""

Light is a metaphor for consciousness in all spiritual traditions. "Motion and rest" suggest the qualifies of nature, activity and inertia, and which our minds and bodies are constantly involved in. When we trace them to their source, however, we discover the primal cause, conscious energy, what Jesus referred to as the Father.

Compare this with *Yoga-sutra* IV.34: "Thus the supreme state of Absolute Freedom manifests while the qualities reabsorb themselves into Nature, having no more purpose to serve the Self. Or (from another angle), the power of pure consciousness settles in its own pure nature."[14]

And with:

> "The luminaries Fire, Sun and Moon
> Their luminousness received by Grace of Divine Light;
> The Light that gave that Light
> Is a Mighty Light of Effulgence Immense;
> That Light dispelling my darkness,
> In me stood into oneness suffused".
> (*Thirumandiram*, verse 2683)

> "I have known the Lord from days bygone
> But the Celestials knew Him not,
> Doubt-tossed are they;
> The Lord is the Light,
> In my fleshy body as Prana pulsates
> If I know Him not, who else will?"
> (*Thirumandiram,* verse 1797)

Jesus urges his hearers to become one with who he truly is by deeply imbibing the teachings from his mouth:

Saying 108:

"Whoever drinks from my mouth will become like me; I myself shall become that person, and the hidden things will be revealed to that person."

When we do so, we go beyond the words and realize their source, our true identity, which like that of Jesus, is Divine. Words divide. They make distinctions between this and that; this belief versus that belief. Consequently, religion itself becomes an agent for division, leading to conflict. Spirituality is untainted by any division. To become spiritual is to transcend the divisions of names, forms and beliefs. As long as we limit ourselves to believing in words, however, we will never see the living Presence, immanent everywhere, within and without.

On Entering into the Kingdom of Heaven

The kingdom of Heaven is the state of consciousness known in Yoga as *samadhi,* which is sometimes translated as "cognitive absorption" or "the breathless state of communion with the Lord."[15] To enter it requires that one first acquire the wisdom (*jnana*) of who one truly is, and then pass through a process of purification, wherein one gradually ceases to identify with the body and the mind. Ignorance of one's true identity, the eternal Self, the soul, cannot be dissolved, however, merely by a change of opinion or philosophy, but only gradually as one expands one's consciousness and enters repeatedly into the state of *samadhi.* In *samadhi,* one becomes aware of what is aware. "The supreme Self shines in undisturbed calmness." *Yoga-Sutra* I.47[16] It is a state of innocence, in which one sees the face we had before we were born.

Saying 22:

Jesus saw some babies nursing. He said to His followers, "These nursing babies are like those who enter the Kingdom."

They said to him, "Then shall we enter the Kingdom as babies?"

Jesus said to them, "When you make the two into one, and when you make the inner like the outer and the outer like the inner, and the upper like the lower, and when you make male and female into a single one, so that the male will not be male nor the female be female, when you make eyes in place of an eye, a hand in place of a hand, a foot in place of a foot, an image in place of an image, then you will enter (the Kingdom)."

In other words, we can enter into "the Kingdom of Heaven" when we go beyond the divisions and distinctions created by the mind, when we transcend the pairs of opposites, when we realize that which exists behind the thought of "I," the thought of "eye," referred to by Jesus, that which is the Witness to our seeing and walking. Jesus is referring to the realization of the Seer, as distinct from the Seen. This pure, attributeless consciousness is referred to in Yoga and the *Samkhya* philosophy underlying Yoga, as the Self. Its realization is *samadhi*, what Jesus referred to as entering into "the Kingdom of Heaven."

The Gospel of Thomas reveals Jesus as both a wandering sage, dispensing Gnostic wisdom, shaking his listeners out of their habitual mind frames, and as an initiating *Guru*, who reveals to the most worthy the realization of their true identify with the Supreme.

"The Jesus of the churches is founded upon the literary character, Jesus, composed by Mark... The living Jesus, portrayed by Thomas, never the man who was crucified nor the God who was resurrected, is himself the fullness of where once we were. And that surely is one of the effects of the Gospel of Thomas, which is to undo the Jesus of the New Testament and return us to an earlier Jesus."[17] In doing so it reminds us that by the careful application of the wisdom of Jesus, we will find the face we had before the world was made.

Was Jesus a Gnostic?

Given that what Jesus really said is now authenticated by the consensus of modern critical scholarship, and in light of the Gospel of Thomas, there is little doubt that Jesus used much of the language of the Gnostics. But there is little or no evidence that he was part of any Gnostic community. The authenticated parables, aphorisms and sage retorts of Jesus corresponded to several, but not all of the characteristics of Gnostics cited above:

- A radical cosmic dualism that rejects this world and all that belongs to it: the body is a prison from which the soul longs to escape. While Jesus was a homeless person, and did not marry, rejected his family, and spent much time in solitude in the wilderness, he also welcomed children, responded with compassion to the most common forms of human suffering, such as fever, blindness, paralysis, and mental illness, and wept when he realized his people had rejected him.[18] He never referred to the world as evil, nor encouraged others to escape from it.

- A distinction between the unknown transcendent true God and the Creator, or Demiurge, commonly identified with the God of the Hebrew Bible: Both in the Gospel of Thomas and in the recently discovered *Gospel of Judas,* this distinction is made by the writers, who are quoting Jesus. But the Creator God is not described as being evil.

- The belief that the human race is essentially akin to the divine, being a spark of heavenly light imprisoned in a material body: statements by Jesus in the Gospel of Thomas reflect this Gnostic view to some extent. Jesus, for example, speaks as the redeemer coming from God. He reminds his followers of their forgetfulness and tells them they are in need of enlightenment (Thomas 28). He deprecates the world. (Thomas 21.6, 27.1, 56.1, 80.1-2, 110, 111.3) He reminds people of their origin (Thomas 49) and shows them how to escape from this world. (Thomas 50) He also speaks of his own return to the place from which he has come.

- A myth, often narrating a pre-mundane fall, to account for the present human predicament: Jesus did not refer to any cosmological myths about the origins of the world, nor any which would explain its present condition, nor did he speak of his own personal visions.

- The saving knowledge by which deliverance is effected and the Gnostic awakened to recognition of his or her true nature and heavenly origin. The primary message of Jesus is how to find the Kingdom of Heaven, which is both imminent and transcendent.

Throughout his authenticated sayings, he refers to the search for it. (See Thomas 26 and 94 for examples)

How is One to Realize the Gnosis, the Saving Knowledge?

Many of the aphorisms and parables of Jesus and the Gnostics direct the listener to search for that saving knowledge, but refrain from telling anyone how to search. Discovering that for oneself is, apparently the first step toward self-knowledge.

Saying 6:

His disciples questioned Him and said to Him, "Do you want us to fast? How shall we pray? Shall we give alms? What diet shall we observe?" Jesus said, "Do not tell lies, and do not do what you hate because all things are disclosed before heaven. For there is nothing hidden that will not be revealed, and there is nothing covered that will remain undisclosed."

Jesus' ironic answer turns his listeners back upon themselves. Who but oneself can judge when one is lying or what one hates? For example, when we worry we are meditating on what we do not want, i.e., "what you hate." How can we stop doing this? The first step is to become aware. The next step is to exercise our will. Becoming aware means witnessing the reactions of the mind and body; it also means adopting a new perspective, realizing that you are not your mind or body, but that they are vehicles in which you are traveling through space and time. Then one can stand back as the Witness, and observed in a detached manner, their habitual movements. Noticing these, one can begin to exercise one's willpower, and think, speak and act only after reflection, what is edifying and necessary only.

Several of the texts found at Nag Hammadi along with the Gospel of Thomas do describe techniques of spiritual discipline designed to bring the saving Gnosis. *Zostrianos*, the longest of these texts, tells how one spiritual master attained enlightenment, implicitly setting out a program for others to follow. This included initially purifying oneself of physical desires, then calming the "chaos of the mind," sitting in meditation, and then as a result, gaining a vision of the "perfect child" a "divine presence," and subsequently of "the Eternal Light."

Another Gnostic text, *Discourse on the Eighth and the Ninth,* gives more specific instructions, including the chanting of sacred words and vowels, which lead one into ecstatic states, and the cultivation of mental silence, wherein all knowledge is gained. In the *Allogenes* (Greek, "another race" or "a stranger"), the spiritually mature person becomes a stranger to the world through progressive stages of Gnosis, using prayer, chanting, meditation and retreats. Ultimately, while one discovers the "good within" according to one's capacity, one cannot attain knowledge about the Unknown God.[19]

In 1 Corinthians 2.6, the Apostle Paul also claims to initiate worthy disciples into a secret wisdom:

"Yet among the mature we do impart wisdom, although it is not a wisdom of this age or of the rulers of this age, who are doomed to pass away. But we impart a secret and hidden wisdom of God, which God decreed before the ages for our glorification."

Followers of the second century Gnostic leader Valentinus, who was a disciple of Theudas, a disciple of Paul, say that their own Gospels and revelations disclose those secret teachings.[20]

But most of the Gnostic teachings on spiritual discipline remained, on principle, unwritten; for anyone can read what is written down. Gnostic teachers reserved their instructions for secret initiations, sharing it only verbally, to ensure each candidate's suitability to receive it. Such instruction required each teacher to take responsibility for highly select, individualized attention to each candidate, and it required the candidate, in turn, to devote energy and time - often years - to the process. Such a program would appeal only to a few. As such, the spiritual perspectives and methods of instruction did not lend themselves to mass religion. It was no match for the highly effective system of organization of the Catholic Church, which expressed a unified religious perspective based on the New Testament Canon, offered a creed requiring the member to confess only the simplest essentials of faith, and celebrated rituals as simple and profound as baptism and the *Eucharist*. (Greek, "communion") These elements are common to all Christian denominations, and largely explain why organized Christianity has survived to this day.[21]

However, it still begs the question: "How is one to realize the Gnosis, the saving Knowledge?" and to do so today. Is the Gnosis still accessible? What is the Gnosis that the sayings in the Gospel of Thomas are pointing to? Before attempting to answer these questions, let us first turn to what modern research has discovered about the teachings of Jesus.

CHAPTER 4

Early Christianity: the Formation of the Church and its Dogma

To understand the wisdom teachings of Jesus Christ, it is instructive to trace the history of Christianity from the period when he lived to the time when it became the Roman state religion and the twenty seven books of the New Testament canon were ratified at the Synod of Hippo, at the end of the fourth century. The various early forms of Christianity which competed with each other will be surveyed and compared. This will help bring into focus the discussion, in subsequent chapters, of what Jesus said and did not say, and why the teachings of Jesus have been obscured. Bear in mind, throughout this chapter, that the particular form of Christianity that eventually triumphed over the others was forged in large part by political and cultural forces that had little to do with the teachings of Jesus Himself. Consider also what Christianity might have become had one of the other early forms of Christianity been victorious.

The Dead Sea Scrolls and the Essenes

The Dead Sea Scrolls were first discovered early in 1947. A shepherd, looking for his goat, stumbled upon a series of caves at Qumram, in the cliffs above the Dead Sea, and inside found a group of sealed pottery jars, each about two feet tall, some of which were broken. Inside each jar were leather scrolls covered in an ancient text. While he admitted to finding seven scrolls, there were others which have not been passed onto the authorities. After several years, scholars began to link the scrolls to the early Christian community. The first to do so was Professor André Dupont-Sommer, of the Sorbonne Univeristy in Paris. He drew parallels between the leader of the Essene community at Qumram, in the first century B.C., the "Teacher of Righteousness," never named, but described in the Habbakuk scroll, believed to be divine, put to death by his enemies and expected to rise from the dead, and Jesus. Judaism had formed a whole theology centered around this suffering Messiah, long before Jesus was even born.

Linen taken from the cave where the scrolls were found was carbon dated in 1951 to a period of 33 C.E. plus or minus two hundred years. Coins were also found in the caves: all of them from the beginning of the Christian era to 70 C.E., the end of the Jewish war.

Archaelogical studies of the caves at Qumram has revealed that the scrolls were probably not written there, but brought there from Jerusalem. The site was probably a farm, not a monastery.

In 1958 another scroll was discovered in one of the caves. In it, a text referred to a figure who "will be called son of God." The usage of the term "son of God" until then had been thought to pertain only to Jesus. Its discovery linked the scrolls to the formation of early Christianity. All of the above demonstrated that the Dead Sea scrolls came from a group of messianic Jews, with a theology which was very similar to that of early Christianity. However, Christianity broke away from Judaism and the law.

The discovery and analysis of the scrolls has a direct impact on the central tenets of Nicene Christianity: first, that Jesus Christ was unique, and secondly that he was divine and that therefore supersedes the Jewish law in importance. Regarding the first challenge to Christian Nicene theology, the scrolls provide sufficient evidence that the New Testament and Jesus emerged from a preexisting messianic Jewish context. So, Christianity is not based upon a unique event in history, but emerged from an existing movement that even used the term "son of God," which until the scrolls discovery was thought to be unknown in Judaism and fundamental to the founding of Christianity.

The second challenge, which the scrolls have made to Nicene Christianity occurs because the scrolls call into question the theological unity of the Gospels. They reveal the clash between James, the brother of Jesus and the leader of the Jerusalem messianic community, described in the Book of Acts, which like the Essenian community which produced the Dead Sea scrolls, stressed the need for adherence to Jewish law - and Paul who maintained that one is saved by one's belief in the divinity of Jesus, as one savior, and freedom from adherence to the Jewish law.

As we will see below, these issues reappeared in subsequent centuries as various early sects of Christianity sought to answer the question "Who is Jesus?" and "How does one enter the Kingdom of Heaven?"[1]

Early Christian Historical Sources

During the first decades following the crucifixion of Jesus, his followers multiplied in a large number of diverse churches (Greek *ekklesias* – "assemblies") of Christians. The fifth book in the New Testament, Acts of the Apostles, written around 80 C.E. by the same anonymous author as the Gospel of Luke, provides the only continuous record of the expansion of Christianity during the thirty years following the crucifixion of Jesus. In particular it traces the travels and activities of Paul, and end with his speeches and imprisonment in Rome. However, it says relatively little about other apostles. It provides a hinge between the four Gospels and the letters of Paul in the New Testament.[2] But scholars today recognize that it cannot be used uncritically to provide a historical basis for understanding the relationship between orthodoxy and heresy, and the competing "Christianities" lead by Paul, Peter, and other early apostles and their followers. Analysis of this book, the Acts of the Apostles, and comparison with other New Testament books reveals that it was driven as much by a theological agenda as by a concern for historical accuracy.[3]

There was not another Christian historian for another two and a half centuries. Eusebius, an early fourth century historian, provides our best source of history of the early Christian Church in his ten volume *Church History*. The beliefs of the various Christian assemblies were as diverse as there were answers to the questions: Who was Jesus? Was he God? And must one fulfill the Jewish Law to enter the Kingdom of Heaven? Jesus Himself anticipated the ensuing debate when he asked his disciples: "Who do men say that I am?" (Luke 9.18) And they answered, "John the Baptist;" but others say, Elijah; and others, that one of the old prophets has risen! And He said to them, "But who do you say that I am?" And Peter answered, "The Christ of God." And then Jesus commanded them to tell this to no one. (Luke 19-21)

But what did this mean? There were many divergent views among early Christian churches. Each had their own teachings, based upon their answer to the above questions. They agreed however, that while Jesus was a Jew, his teachings were for Gentiles as well.

Paulism

Paul was the most important early Christian missionary to the Gentiles. Gentiles worshipped many gods. To accept the salvation of Jesus, they had to renounce their former gods, he taught, and accept only the God of Israel and Jesus his Son, whose death, and resurrection, would bring them salvation from God. But did this mean that they had to become Jewish, and observe the Jewish Law, given by the Jewish God? According to this Law, His people must set themselves apart in distinctive ways, for example, by keeping the seventh day holy, by following kosher dietary laws (such as avoiding pork and shellfish), and by receiving the sign of their covenant with God (circumcision of the male organ). So, did a Gentile first have to become Jewish in order to become a Christian? Some of the earliest disciples of Jesus, including Peter, believed that one did. Paul's letters in rebuttal indicate that there were outspoken, sincere, and active Christian leaders who passionately disagreed with him on this, and considered Paul's views to be a corruption of the true message of Christ. Paul, on the other hand, believed that for Gentiles to adopt the ways of

Judaism meant to call into question the salvation God had provided by the death of Jesus. One is made right with God only by faith in Jesus' death and resurrection, not by following any of the deeds prescribed by the Jewish Law. In Galatians 2:11-14, in which Paul attacks these Christian missionaries, he even indicates that he had a public encounter with Peter over this issue in the city of Antioch. He disagreed with one of Jesus' closest disciple on the matter. Unfortunately, history has not preserved the response of Peter. Paul does not indicate the outcome of the public altercation, leading to the widely held suspicion that this was one debate that Paul lost, at least in the eyes of those who observed it. The debate raged even among the authors of the canonical Gospels. The author of Matthew, the most "Jewish" of the four Gospels, alone quotes Jesus in support of this position:

"Do not think that I have come to destroy the Law and the prophets; I did not come to destroy but to fulfill. For truly I say to you, until heaven and earth pass away, not the smallest letter or the smallest stroke of a letter will pass away from the Law until all has taken place. Whoever lets loose one of the least of these commandments and teaches others to do likewise will be called least in the kingdom of heaven. For I say to you that if your righteousness does not exceed that of the scribes and Pharisees, you will not enter the Kingdom of Heaven." (Matthew 5:17-20)

It is hard to imagine Paul agreeing with the author of the Gospel of Matthew, or even with Peter. After both Paul and Peter died, advocates of their respective positions on the Law and the person of Jesus developed their views. Those advocating Paul's position eventually won, and are referred to by scholars today as the "proto-orthodox." They eventually defined Christian orthodoxy in a series of creeds, or doctrines of faith, after centuries of debate. Then their adherents systematically suppressed as heretical the teachings of their opponents. Consequently, there were, indeed, many "lost Christianities." A study of their beliefs and history helps to reveal the issues which eventually helped to define Christianity as we know it today.

The Roman Empire contained religions of all kinds. This multiplicity bred respect and for the most part, tolerance. With the possible exception of Judaism, the worship of the gods never involved accepting or making doctrinally acceptable claims about a god. There were no creeds devised to proclaim the true nature of the gods and their interactions with the world, no "orthodoxy" (right beliefs) or "heresy" (false beliefs). What mattered were traditionally sanctioned acts of worship.[4] But as soon as some Christians began proclaiming that salvation or right standing with God depended upon a profession of Jesus as one's savior, then this new religion became exclusivist. One was saved if one professed one's faith in Jesus as savior; one was damned if one did not. This then required that Christians decide upon the content of their faith, and this raised endless questions and issues. Once the importance of what one believed determined one's salvation or damnation for eternity, the debates began. They were long, hard fought, and often ugly.

Early Doctrinal Issues

Among the most important questions and issues debated were the following: "What does one need to believe about Jesus? That he was a man? An angel? A divine being? Was he a god? Was he God? If Jesus is God and God is God, how can we be monotheists who believe in one God? And if the Spirit is God, too, then don't we have three Gods? Or is Jesus God the Father himself come to earth for the salvation of the world? If so, then when Jesus prayed to God, was he speaking to himself? And what was it about Jesus that brought salvation? His public teachings which if followed provide the way to eternal life? His secret teachings, meant only for the spiritually elite, whose proper understanding is the key to unity with God? His way of life, which is to be modeled by followers who, like him, must give up all they have for the sake of the Kingdom? His death on the cross? Did he die on the cross? Why would he die on the cross?"[5]

Among the most prominent early Christian churches involved in these debates were the Docetists, the Ebionites, the Marcionites, the Gnostics and the proto-Orthodox.

Docetism

The term "Docetism" is derived from the Greek word *doceo* – "appear" or "seem." Two forms of this belief were widely known.[6] According to some Docetists, Jesus was so completely divine that he could not possibly be human. God could not have a material body, and could not have suffered pain and died. So, Jesus only "appeared" to be a flesh-and-blood human being. The second type of Docetists made a distinction between Jesus, who was a real flesh and blood human being, and the Christ, a divine being who, as God, could not experience pain and death. In their view, the divine Christ descended from heaven as a dove and entered into the body of Jesus at the time of his baptism. This divine Christ remained with and empowered Jesus to perform miracles and deliver radical teachings, until just before his death, when it departed. That is why, according to them, Jesus cried out, "My God, my God, why have you forsaken me?" (Mark 15.34) or as it is more literally translated: "Why have you left me behind?" For these Docetists, God, the divine Christ, had left Jesus behind by re-ascending to heaven, leaving Jesus to die on the cross.[7]

Ebionitism

According to these early Jewish Christians, Jesus was a flesh and blood human being, born out of the sexual union of his parents, Joseph and Mary. But because he had kept God's law perfectly and so was the most righteous man on earth, God had adopted him as his son, and given him a special mission. He was to be a perfect sacrifice to atone for humanity's sins, in fulfillment of God's promise to the Jews, his people, in their Scriptures. While the Ebionites continued to follow all other Jewish practices, such as observing the Sabbath, circumcision and eating only kosher food, they no longer participated in the ritualistic sacrifices of animals. Many were vegetarians, as was John the Baptist, and evidently, Jesus, his successor. They considered Paul to be their arch enemy, because he taught that one could find salvation from God, not by keeping the Law, but by believing in Jesus as one's savior. They claimed that their views were authorized by the original disciples, especially Peter and James (the brother of Jesus and head of the Jerusalem church).[8]

Marcionites

At the opposite end of the theological spectrum, but living at the same time (the second to third centuries) were the Marcionites, who rejected everything Jewish. They were followers of the second century evangelist and theologian, Marcion, one of the most important Christian theologians and writers of the early centuries. We know more about them, because the proto-Orthodox (the followers of the teachings of Paul) took them more seriously. Few Gentiles were attracted to Jewish Law, with all of its restrictions, nor to surgical circumcision of their penises. But the Marcionites had a religion which was highly attractive to pagans and Gentiles. The Marcionites rejected Jewish Law and the Jewish God. Marcion was born around 100 C.E. on the southern shore of the Black Sea. His father was the bishop of the Church there. He became a wealthy merchant, and went to Rome, where he donated a huge sum of money to the Church there. He called the first council of Church leaders there, where he presented his views.

Marcion was attracted by the writings of Paul, and in particular to one passage in Galatians where Paul makes a distinction between the Law of the Jews and the Gospel of Christ. It was faith in Christ, not works according to the Law, which would bring one to God. Marcion made this distinction the foundation of his teachings. The Gospel is the good news of deliverance, and it includes love, mercy, grace, forgiveness, reconciliation, redemption, and life. The Law is the bad news that makes the Gospel necessary: it includes strict commandments, as well as sin, guilt, judgment, damnation, and death. How could the same God be responsible for both? How could an angry, vengeful God of the Jews be the loving, merciful God of Jesus? Marcion argued that these attributes could not belong to the same God. There must be two Gods: the God of the Jews as described in the Old Testament, and the God of Jesus, as described in the writings of Paul.

Everything else in Marcion's theology derives logically from this conclusion. Like the Docetists, he taught that Jesus did not belong to this material world, but only appeared to be human. He wrote two literary works: The first was the *Antithesis* (Greek – "setting opposite"), a commentary on the Bible, in which he draws pointed contrasts between the two Gods. His second work was the first Christian Canon of Scripture, consisting of the Gospel of Luke, ten of the twelve letters of Paul (except 1 and 2 Timothy), and Titus. His Canon probably spurred subsequent Christian leaders like Irenaeus to begin to assemble what, decades later, became the New Testament. Paul was the one predecessor he could trust to understand the radical claims of the Gospel. Jesus' disciples, themselves followers of the Jewish God, continued to interpret Jesus' words, deeds, and death in light of their understanding of Judaism. So, Jesus revealed himself and the truth of his Gospel to Paul, in order to start afresh, to reveal the truth of his gospel, and to confront the disciples Peter and James, as seen in the letter to the Galatians.

Marcion's views were rejected by the Church leaders in Rome, so he returned to Asia Minor, where he became tremendously successful in propagating his views and founding churches. For many centuries they were the original and dominant form of Christianity in Asia Minor.[9]

The Gnostics

Gnosis is the Greek word for knowledge. There was not one "Gnosticism" but many. Its origins were probably in the Jewish apocalyptic traditions up to the 4th century B.C. as well as Persia, Babylonia and perhaps India. Its adherents were members of many diverse Christian churches, but considered themselves in possession of special knowledge by which they could return to the Kingdom of God. In Chapter 2, their chief characteristics were discussed. By way of summary, these included a rejection of the material world, a distinction between the unknown transcendent true God and the creator God, commonly identified with the God of the Hebrew Bible, the belief that humans are a spark of heavenly light imprisoned in a material body, myth, often narrating a primordial fall, to account for the present human predicament, and saving knowledge (*gnosis*) by which the Gnostic is awakened to recognition of his or her true nature and heavenly origin.[10]

The classic period of Gnosticism is the second century C.E. with such figures as Basilides and Valentinus, and the latter's disciples Ptolemy and

Heracleon, but this was the culmination of a long development. According to the various Gnostic myths, the one unknowable God, Who is totally perfect, incapable of description and beyond attributes, generated a divine realm from Himself, and from it other divine entities, called *Aeons* (Greek – "the ever-existing"), which in turn produced their own entities (thought, eternality, life, etc.), until there was an entire realm, sometimes called the *Pleroma* (Greek – "Fullness"). The diverse Gnostic myths are designed to show not only how this Pleroma came into existence but how the world we live in came into being and how we ourselves came to be here. They share a belief that this material world is the result of a disruption in the Pleroma, a catastrophe in the Cosmos, created by the creator God. This world we live in was not the idea or creation of the One True God, but the result of a cosmic disaster, and that within some humans there resides a spark of the divine that needs to be liberated in order to return to its real home. Christ provides the knowledge necessary for salvation.

This is knowledge of ourselves – "Knowledge of who we were and what we have become, of where we were and where we have been made to fall, of where we are hastening and from where we are being redeemed, of what birth is and what rebirth." (Theodotos, according to Clement of Alexandria's *Excerpts from Theodotus*, 78.2)

This knowledge is secret, reserved for an elite who are able to penetrate its subtleties, and brought by one who has come down from the divine realm to remind us of our true identity, our true origin, and our true destiny. This divine emissary has been sent not by the creator God of the Jewish Bible, but by the true God, to reveal to us the true state of things and the means of escape. Those who receive and understand and accept these teachings will be "Gnostics," those "in the know."[11]

Valentinus claims that, besides receiving the Christian tradition that all believers hold in common, he has received from Theudas, a disciple of Paul, initiation into a secret doctrine of God. Paul himself taught this secret wisdom, he says, not to everyone and not publicly, but only to a select few whom he considered to be spiritually mature. Valentinus offers to initiate those who are mature into his wisdom, since not everyone is able to comprehend it.[12]

Some scholars suspect that Gnostic Christians did not treat their myths as literal descriptions of the past, in the way modern fundamentalist Christians might treat the opening chapters of Genesis. Today, most non fundamentalist Christians agree that Genesis contains mythical and legendary accounts. One does not have to believe in a literal six day creation, or that Adam and Eve were historical persons to belong to modern non fundamentalist Christian churches.

For the proto-Orthodox, the Gnostics were the enemies within the Church, not outside it. For, "the Gnostics did not deny the validity of the proto-Orthodox doctrinal claims per se; instead, they reinterpreted them in a way that they considered more spiritual and insightful. They could confess the proto-Orthodox creeds, read the proto-Orthodox Scriptures, accept their Sacraments. But all these things were understood differently for Gnostics, based upon their fuller insight into their real meaning, a fuller insight available to them because of their superior knowledge (*gnosis*) of divine truth."[13]

For the Gnostics, it is not the death of Christ on the cross that brings us salvation, but the living Christ. For the body is just a shell, belonging to the creator of this world. Salvation does not come in the body, but by escaping it.

The Proto-Orthodox

Only one form of Christianity emerged as victorious. It was influenced by all of the others. In fact, its opposition to alternative perspectives drove proto-Orthodox Christians to the views they did, and to define them in creeds and dogma. We owe to the proto-Orthodox the most familiar features of what is considered as Christianity today: four Gospels only, twenty-seven books in the New Testament, and included in this Canon of Orthodox Scripture, the Old Jewish Bible. We owe to proto-Orthodoxy, as well the church hierarchy, a set of doctrinal beliefs (Christ as both fully God and fully man; the sacred Trinity: Father, Son and Holy

Spirit) and the sacraments of baptism and the Eucharist, marriage and death.

Ignatius, Bishop of Antioch, whose writings at the beginning of the second century C.E. are considered to be among the most important proto-Orthodox works, emphasized the importance of martyrdom, "to attain God," and to differentiate true and false believers, as well as the authority of the bishop, church order and structure.

The author of the book *1 Clement*, probably the third bishop of Rome around 90-100 C.E. argued in a letter to the church of Corinth, whose leaders had been thrown out by a rival faction, that the leaders must be reinstated because of "Apostolic Succession." God sent Christ, who chose the twelve Apostles, and the twelve Apostles chose church leaders, and those leaders in turn handpicked their successors. (Chapters 42, 44) The deposed leaders of the Corinth church stood in a lineage chosen by the Apostles, and to oppose them meant to set oneself against the Apostles, Christ and God. So, Tertullian and Irenaeus, early proto-Orthodox theologians, also used "Apostolic Succession" to counter any claims by Gnostics or others to the truth. "No one except the bishops appointed by the heirs of Christ could possibly be right about the precious truths of the faith."[14] This argument overlooked the fact that already in the second century, there were bishops, including the bishops of Rome, who were themselves declared heretical by well-intentioned proto-Orthodox theologians. In using this argument, Tertullian named only two churches which could trace their direct lineage to apostles: Smyrna (whose bishop Polycarp was appointed by the apostle John) and Rome, whose bishop Clement was appointed by Peter. But we also know that Valentinus was a disciple of Theudas, who was in turn a disciple of Paul; and the Gnostic Basilides was a disciple of Glaukia, a disciple of Peter.[15] "Obey the bishop" was the argument used by the proto-Orthodox, with effect, and was based upon the assumption that if the right people are in charge, they will know what to do.

There had not always been this emphasis on church hierarchy. When Paul wrote his letters to various churches, he did not write them to church leaders, but to the church congregation as a whole. This was because there was no person in charge. Paul's churches, as evidenced in 1 Corinthians itself, were organized as charismatic communities, directed by the Spirit of God, who gave each member a special gift (Greek: *charisma*) to assist them to live and function together as a communal body, gifts of teaching, prophesying, giving, leading and so on. (1 Cor. 12)

After Paul's death, an aspiring author in one of his churches wrote the Pastoral Epistles (1 and 2 Timothy and Titus) in Paul's name, and addressed them to the pastors of troubled churches. Then came the work, *1 Clement*, from the bishop of Rome. Within a century, Christians became accustomed to opposing "aberrant" forms of Christianity by arguing that the bishops of the leading churches in the world could trace their lineage back through their personal predecessors to the Apostles themselves, who appointed them.

Unlike today, in the ancient Roman world there was a general distrust of any philosophy or religion that was new. The "old" was appreciated and respected. Nothing "new" could be true, for if it was true, why was it not known long ago? Why was it not known by the Greeks: Homer, Plato or Aristotle? In seeking to convert Gentiles or pagans to Christianity, Christians devised a strategy which would enable them to avoid this objection. Even though Jesus had lived only decades or a century ago, they argued, Christianity is based upon a religion which is much older than the Greeks: the Old Testament. They interpolated statements into the New Testament to show that God had predicted the coming of Jesus in the writings of Moses and the prophets. By taking over the Jewish scriptures, and making them their own, Christian evangelists overcame the biggest single objection that pagans had with regards to the appearance of this new religion.[16]

Proto-orthodox writers also followed the strategy of basing their authority on Scriptural sources. As described above, they sought religious legitimacy in the eyes of Gentiles by pointing to the Jewish Old Testament as their basis. They claimed that they were the true inheritors of the covenant of the Jewish God with Moses. However, while embracing the Jewish Scriptures, at the same time they rejected Judaism and the Jews. There was no need to follow the Jewish Law, because the true believers in Christ were saved by their faith. Ignatius argued that Christ is himself the point of the Jewish Bible. This became the trademark of non-Jewish Christians. The Epistle of Barnabas, written about 130 C.E. was the most famous proto-Orthodox text to exhibit this strategy. It also attacked the Jews, and set the stage for other increasingly anti-Semitic writings, who blamed the Jews for the death and crucifixion of Jesus. All this led to great tensions with Jewish neighbors, who thought that Christians were trying to usurp their traditions, while not even keeping its laws.

Proto-Orthodoxy at first embraced direct revelation from God, including the Book of Revelation. After much debate, it was finally included in the Canon of the New Testament. But soon, problems with this became apparent: How can one determine whether a "prophecy" comes from God or not? What if it does not agree with Scripture? But if the Scripture is the key to everything, why does one need prophecy at all? Also, how can divine teaching be controlled by the emerging church if it is a matter of personal inspiration?

But the respect which the proto-Orthodox showed for the Jewish scriptures did not extend to philosophical works. They argued that "truth precedes error," and therefore, as Irenaeus argued, if philosophy could reveal the truth about God, what was the point of sending Christ into the world? (*Against Heresies* 2.14.6-7) Hippolytus of Rome devoted the first four volumes of his ten volume *Refutation of All Heresies* to showing that heresy derives from Greek philosophical tradition. Tertullian completely rejects the infusion of philosophy into the truth of the Christian gospel; as he famously asks, "What indeed has Athens to do with Jerusalem? What concord is there between the Academy and the Church? What between heretics and Christians?" in *Prescription*, 7.[17]

The proto-Orthodox strategy also involved emphasis on the notion of "unity" on all levels: between God and his creation, between God and Jesus, between Jesus and Christ, and finally the unity of the church. Division therefore is caused by heretics. Truth is also one; it cannot be contradictory or at odds with itself. Therefore those who would cause division in the church are not speaking the truth, was their argument.

The most important defining marker separating the proto-Orthodox from others, however, was the development of the doctrine of Christ as fully God and fully man, and the doctrine of the Trinity: one God in three persons, distinct in number but equal in substance. Debates which resulted in these doctrines began to emerge soon after the resurrection of Christ. Was he human or divine? Did he suffer? Did God suffer? If Jesus was Divine, then there is not One God. How can anyone be his own Father? Who was Jesus praying to? Ignatius, and later Origin, (184-254 AD) the most learned, prolific and famous theologian of the first three centuries, sought to solve the problem. Origen wrote more than a thousand books, supported by his wealthy Alexandria, Egypt, patron Ambrose, and an army of stenographers and scribes. Origin's theology was biblically based from beginning to end. God was the Creator of all things, including Christ. Christ is God's Word made flesh; Christ is God, one with the Father, distinct in person, but equal in substance. His key conclusion was that Christ is equal with God by the transference of God's being; ultimately, he is subordinate to God and is "less than the Father."[18]

Ironically, Origen was later condemned for this innovative resolution of the relationship between God and Christ when orthodox thinkers in later centuries refined their categories and came to reject any notion of Christ's subordination to God, which to them implied that he was not equal in essence to God.

The Cultural and Political Factors Which Favored the Proto-Orthodox

How was it that the proto-Orthodox established itself as the dominant form of Christianity? We have observed, above, several factors which favored their success:

- They claimed ancient roots for their religion.
- They rejected the practices of contemporary Judaism, allowing their form of Christianity to become a universal faith, attractive and feasible for the majority of the people of the ancient world.
- They stressed a church hierarchy, unlike the Gnostics (who believed everyone in their community had equal access to the secret

liberating knowledge). The church hierarchy was invested with an authority that was used to determine what was to be believed, how worship and church affairs were to be conducted, and which books were to be accepted as scriptural authorities.

- They were in constant communication with one another, and were determined to establish their faith as a worldwide communion.

All of the above involve written texts. So, the battle for supremacy turned upon the battle over texts. The canonization of the twenty seven books of the New Testament marked the victory of the proto-Orthodox.[19]

But as Elaine Pagels in her book *The Gnostic Gospels* has concluded: "Yet the majority of Christians, Gnostic and orthodox, like religious people of every tradition, concerned themselves with ideas primarily as expressions or symbols of religious experience. Such experience remains the source and testing ground of all religious ideas (as, for example, a man and a woman are likely to experience differently the idea that God is masculine). Gnosticism and orthodoxy, then, articulated very different kinds of human experience; I suspect that they appealed to different types of persons."[20]

As the Gnostic scholar Arthur Darby Nock has stated: "Gnosticism involves no recoil from society, but a desire to concentrate on inner well being."[21] The Gnostic pursued an essentially solitary path. According to the *Gospel of Thomas*, Jesus praises this solitude. "Blessed are the solitary and chosen, for you will find the Kingdom. For you are from it, and to it you will return."[22] This solitude comes from the Gnostic's insistence on the primacy of immediate experience. No one else can tell another which way to go, what to do, or how to act. The Gnostic could not accept on faith what others said, except as a provisional measure, until one found one's own path. While they may rely on the testimony of others initially, when they become mature, they discover their own immediate relationship with the truth itself. Only on the basis of immediate experience could one create the poems, vision accounts, myths, and hymns that Gnostics prized as proof that one had actually attained *gnosis*.[23] *The Secret Book of John*, a Gnostic text discovered at Nag Hammadi, speaks of *epinoia*, a higher form of consciousness in which spiritual insights are revealed. This book uses a group of words related to the Greek verb *neoin*, which means "perceive," "think" or "be aware." While God is beyond human understanding, we have powers of consciousness which allow us to glimpse him: *pronoia* (anticipatory awareness), *ennoia*, (internal reflection) and *prognosis* (foreknowledge or intuition).[24] These are comparable to what Patanjali refers to as siddhis, or powers, and to *prajna*, the inspired accompaniments of the state of *samprajnata samadhi*, the fusion of subject and object. In *Yoga-Sutra* I.17 he says: "Distinguished (*samprajnata*) cognitive absorption (*samadhi*) is accompanied by observation, reflecting, rejoicing and awareness of the Self."[25] He further characterizes them as "truth bearing" in I.48. In *Yoga-Sutra* III.5 he tells us "Due to the mastery (of communion) the light of insight arises." Such is not the product of an ordinary intellectual or mental functioning of the mind.

Orthodox Christianity expressed a different kind of experience. Its members were far more concerned with their relationships with other people.

While the Gnostics insisted that humanity's original experience of evil involved internal emotional distress, the Orthodox believed that it came from violation of the natural order, itself essentially "good," primarily in the form of violence towards others. The Orthodox revised the moral code of Moses, which prohibits physical violation of others: murder, stealing and adultery, in terms of Jesus' prohibition against even mental and emotional violence: anger, lust and hatred.[26] Orthodox Christianity's wide popular appeal was termed "perfect because of its unconscious correspondence to the needs and aspirations of ordinary people" by A.D. Nock.[27]

The Gnostics saw the world as evil, and that salvation lies in leaving it. The Orthodox saw the world as "good" and saw Christ not as one who leads souls out of it into enlightenment, but as "fullness of God" come down into human experience - into bodily experience - to make it sacred. The Orthodox also made this ordinary life sacred with the "sacraments" of baptism, the sharing of food in the Eucharist, marriage and death, and all of the major biological events. While the Gnostic saw himself as "one in a thousand" the Orthodox saw themselves as one member of a common human family.

The institutional framework of the proto-Orthodox churches gave to the great majority of people the religious sanction and ethical direction needed for their daily lives. Adapting for its own purposes the model of Roman political and military organization (with bishops, priests and deacons in each church) and gaining in the fourth century imperial support, orthodox Christianity grew increasingly stable and enduring. Gnostic Christianity was no match for the Orthodox faith, either in terms of the Orthodoxy's wide popular appeal or in terms of effective organization. Both have ensured its survival.[28]

The Rule of Faith and Creeds

The proto-Orthodox claim to represent the teachings of the Apostles, the twelve direct disciples of Jesus, resulted in a set of doctrines that expressed for them the true nature of Christianity. By the second century, long before the creation of the Nicene Creed and the Apostles Creed, writers including Irenaeus, Bishop of Lyon, and Tertullian, formulated "*regula fidei.*" (Greek – "rules of faith") These included the basic and fundamental beliefs that according to the proto-Orthodox, all true Christian believers were to subscribe to according to the Apostles. These typically included belief in only one God, the creator of the world, who created everything out of nothing; belief in His Son, Jesus Christ, predicted by the prophets and born of the Virgin Mary; belief in His miraculous life, death, resurrection, and ascension; and belief in the Holy Spirit, Who is present on earth until the end, when there will be a final judgment in which the righteous will be rewarded and the unrighteous condemned to eternal torment. Eventually these rules of faith took the form of creeds, to be recited by converts after baptism and Christian education (*catechisis*), among others.

The creeds were formulated against specific heretical views. They were reactions against doctrinal claims made by groups of Christians who disagreed with them. As a result of the context of their formulation, they are profoundly paradoxical. There is only one God, and He is the creator of all things, but not of the evil and suffering found in his creation. Is Christ God or Man? He is both. If Christ is God and His Father is God, are there two Gods? No, "We believe in one God."[29] The reason for the paradoxes is because the proto-Orthodox felt compelled to fight Marcionism on one side, and Docetists, Ebionites and various types of Gnostics on the other. When one affirms that Jesus is divine, against Ebionites, there is the problem of appearing to be a Docetist. And so one must affirm that he is human, against the Docetist. So the only solution is to affirm both views at once: Jesus is divine and Jesus is human; the Father, Son, and the Spirit are three separate persons, and yet comprise only one God.

The Gospel of John Versus the Gospels of Thomas, Matthew, Mark and Luke

Elaine Pagels, in her book *Beyond Belief: the Secret Gospel of Thomas* demonstrates that the Gospel of John was written by an unknown Jewish scholar, probably living in Ephesus, Asia Minor, at the end of the first century, to specifically refute the Gospel of Thomas and its Gnostic teachings. "What John opposed…includes what the Gospel of Thomas teaches – that God's light shines not only in Jesus but, potentially at least, in everyone. Thomas's gospel encourages the hearer not so much *to believe in Jesus,* as John requires, as to *seek to know God* through one's own, divinely given capacity, since all are created in the image of God. For Christians of later generations, the Gospel of John helped provide a foundation for a unified church, which Thomas, with its emphasis on each person's search for God, did not."[30]

John's Gospel differs from those of Matthew Mark and Luke in several important ways. First, it differs significantly in its account of Jesus' final days. Second, and far more significantly, unlike the other Gospels which present Jesus as God's human servant, or messiah ("anointed one") John suggests that Jesus is "Lord and God" (John 20:28) revealed in human form.[31] It was only after the Gospel of John was appended to the Synoptic Gospels that Christians began to refer to Jesus not as a human being, but as God Himself. Jesus is not merely a messenger for God; Jesus is the message. Third, only the Gospel of John presents a critical and challenging portrait of the disciple Thomas. It is John who invented the character known as "doubting Thomas," as Gregory Riley has pointed out, "perhaps as a way of caricaturing those who revered a teacher - and a version of Jesus' teaching – that he regarded as faithless and false."[32] Fourth, John declares three times at the beginning of his Gospel that the divine light did not penetrate the darkness of the world, and thus God had to send His only begotten Son so that people could see the invisible God. In doing so John rejects Thomas' claim that we have direct access to God through the divine image within us. "He argues that human-kind has no innate capacity to know God. What John's gospel does – and has succeeded ever after in persuading the majority of Christians to do – is to claim that only by believing in Jesus can we find divine truth."[33] Fifth, because this claim is John's primary concern, he offers no ethical or apocalyptic teachings, and does not quote any of the parables of Jesus, as do the other Gospels. This Gospel alone proclaims Jesus' divine identity, speaking in what are referred to as the "I am" sayings. What John does require is that his disciples must believe in Jesus as their Lord God and savior.

Whereas Thomas directs each one to discover the light within, John declares that only Jesus is the light, and only by believing in Jesus can one come to God. In three anecdotes, John alone portrays Thomas as one who doubts Jesus. (John 11.16, John 14.3-4, and John 14.6) Unlike Luke, John refuses to even acknowledge that Thomas was even present when the resurrected Jesus visited the eleven remaining disciples. (John 20.24) At this crucial meeting John claims that Jesus empowered the disciples (but not Thomas) to forgive the sins of others. (John 20.19-23) Finally, by accusing Thomas of being faithless, John claims that Jesus warns everyone that they must believe in him as their Lord God and savior, or face the wrath of God.[34]

One hundred years later, when Irenaeus began to form the New Testament Canon of Gospels, he championed the Gospel of John and rejected that of Thomas. Had the Gospel of Thomas been included or replaced the Gospel of John, Christianity as we now know it would have been far different. Rather than seeking salvation by simply reciting and affirming that Jesus is one's Lord and savior, one would have been initiated into the means of direct access to God through an inner knowledge and light, as described in the "sayings of Jesus," by Christian mystics who had become adept in spiritual practices.

The Formation of the Proto-Orthodox New Testament

The controversies discussed above occurred for the most part after the twenty seven books which eventually became the New Testament were written, that is during a period from 120 C.E. to about 325 C.E. It comes as a shock to most Christians to learn that the Church did not always have the New Testament. The books of Christian scripture did not come down from heaven during the first years or even the first decades after the crucifixion of Jesus. The books that eventually became part of the New Testament Canon were written by a variety of authors over a period of sixty or seventy years, in different places, and for different audiences, beginning with the Letters of Paul during the 50's, then Mark around 65 C.E. and ending with 2 Peter around 120 C.E. Other books were written in the same period, some of them by the same authors. The four Gospels themselves were not written by the four apostles, Matthew, Mark, Luke and John, but by anonymous proto-Orthodox writers. A little later, a flood of books allegedly written by the earliest followers of Jesus, forgeries in the names of the Apostles, began to appear for decades, even centuries, after the Apostles were dead and buried.

While believers may affirm that the selection of the twenty seven books that eventually made it into the New Testament Canon was divinely inspired, this belief generally glazes over the long process of argument and debate, lasting over nearly 300 years, regarding which books to include and which to reject. When it was over, there still was no unanimity.

The first Christian author to advocate the New Testament Canon of twenty seven books was Athanasius, the fourth century bishop of Alexandria. He did so in a letter he wrote in 367 C.E. It was his annual letter to the churches in his diocese in Egypt. These twenty seven books were not officially ratified by the Church however, until the Council of Trent in the mid sixteenth century, and then, this was binding only on Roman Catholics. The Canon of the New Testament came about by a widespread consensus at the end of a long process.

The motivation for this process began with the stress that the Christian religion placed on proper belief. Proper belief required authorities on which to base itself. The Apostles were viewed as authorities of what Jesus said and did. But since they could not be present with Christian congregations everywhere at all times, scriptural texts soon became a critical component to the legitimacy of religious authority. Most of the early Christians were Jews, and they saw Jesus not as the founder of a new religion, but as the fulfillment of the old Jewish religion, whose laws they still followed. The teachings of Jesus are, in large measure, an interpretation of the Jewish Scriptures. Jesus emphasized that the deep intentions of these Laws must be followed, not merely their surface meaning. When most Jews rejected the notion that Jesus was the fulfillment of ancient prophecies, early Christians were motivated to devise their own sacred authoritative scriptures to separate themselves from Jews who refused to accept the interpretations of Jesus. Jesus himself presented his interpretations as authoritative; they were to be the norms for his followers, who considered them to be not only true, but divinely inspired. Soon, not only were Jesus' teachings considered to be sacred Scripture, but also His recorded deeds and the events of His life became so.[35]

The proto-Orthodox claimed all of the Apostles as authorities, but the four Gospels and most of the remaining twenty seven books in the eventual Canon were not written by Apostles. Most scholars agree that the Gospels were written in Greek, in the third person, about Jesus and his companions, by anonymous well educated Christians, during the second half of the first century. None of them were written in the first person, for example: "One day Jesus and I walked to Capernaum…" Recognizing the need for apostolic sources, proto-Orthodox writers falsely attributed these books to Apostles (Matthew and John) and close companions of Apostles (Mark, the secretary of Peter; and Luke the traveling companion of Paul). Other books like James were written by someone who had the same name as the Apostle James. Even the author of the Gospel of John does not claim to have the name "John" nor to be the Apostle John, and probably was not. Others books in the New Testament were written by persons who claimed to be someone they were not: 2 Peter, 1 and 2 Timothy, and Titus, possibly 2 Thessalonians, Colossians and Ephesians, 1 Peter and Jude.[36] The author of Revelations says that his name is "John," (Rev. 1.9) but "John" was a very common name during this period. The author of Revelations does not claim to be John, the son of Zebedee, one of the twelve Apostles of Jesus. In fact, in one scene "John" has a vision of the throne of God surrounded by twenty-four elders who worship Him forever. (Rev. 4:4, 9-10) These twenty-four elders are usually considered to be the twelve apostles and the twelve patriarchs of Israel. But the author gives no indication that he is seeing himself among these twenty-four.[37] Even the early Church historian, Eusebius, a proto-Orthodox Christian, in the early 4th century, who, in his ten volume summary of the writings of the New Testament, created four categories of books (acknowledged, disputed, spurious (forged), and heretical) put Revelations in the category of spurious (forged).[38]

Even though the twenty seven books were all written by 120 AD, quoted passages from them are rare in the letters of church leaders in the first half of the second century. But in the second half of the second century, prophetic movements such as Montanism within proto-Orthodox circles and opposition to heretical forces outside these circles created a demand for an authoritative Canon of Scripture. Montanus and others could claim to have direct revelations from God - claiming that the end of the world was at hand - without the constraint of a written Canon, solid and fixed.

More than anything, however, the formation of an eleven book Canon by Marcion, in the middle of the second century C.E. caused the proto-Orthodox to devise their own Canon. The first of them to do so was Irenaeus, Bishop of Lyon, who chose the four "Gospels" from nearly thirty in his collection, and who added the epistles of Paul, probably in attempt to reclaim Paul from the heretics, as he was a favorite not only of Marcion, but also of the Gnostics. This would also justify his selection of

1 and 2 Timothy and Titus, forged in the name of Paul, which stressed the election of worthy men as bishops and their opposition to the false "gnosis." In the ensuing debates, the proto-Orthodox generally based their choices of what to include in their Canon upon four main criteria:[39]

1. It was ancient: written near the time of Jesus.
2. It was apostolic in authority: it was believed to have been written by an Apostle or at least by a companion of an Apostle. (There was much debate over the books of Hebrews and Revelations in particular because of doubts about the authorship.)
3. It was Catholic: enjoying widespread usage among "established" churches.
4. The most important criteria, by far, was whether the book was consistent with proto-Orthodox views (Peter, for example). If it was not, it could not possibly have been written by an Apostle. On the other hand, the Gospel of Thomas, probably older than the four Gospels, and authored by Thomas the Twin brother of Jesus, was not included because of its Gnostic sayings.

In 393 AD, the Canon proposed by Athanasius was accepted at the Synod of Hippo, in North Africa. Though Rome had not formally ratified it, the Canon of the New Testament was accepted by the Orthodox branches of the Church from this period onwards.

Constantine and the Ecumenical Council of Nicaea

Probably no ten year period was more important to the development of Christianity than 303 to 313 AD, well after the results of the conflicts discussed above had been settled in favor of the proto-Orthodox. The Christians had been persecuted locally, largely by pagans, who believed that their gods were offended when Christians refused to worship them with the prescribed acts of sacrifice. These offenses were widely believed to be the cause of disasters. In 303 the pagan emperor Diocletian in the eastern empire, and Maximian in the western part, both ordered persecution of the Christians. This "Great Persecution" was extensive and lasted for a decade. Then, in 312, the senior emperor, Constantine, began to attribute his military and political ascendancy to the God of the Christians, and to identify himself as a Christian. Once his power base was secure, he became very active in Church affairs, settling controversies, showering support on Christian churches, and organizing the Council of Nicaea, the first ecumenical (Latin *oecumenicus* – "belonging to the whole inhabited world") conference where church leaders from all over the Roman empire were brought together to forge a consensus on major points of faith and practice. It is widely believed that he did so in part because he saw in the Christian Church a means of bringing unity to the empire itself. The proto-Orthodox Christian's belief in One God, one bishop, one Scriptural authority, was consistent with the political needs of the Empire. After Constantine, every emperor except one was Christian. Theodosius I (emperor from 379-95) gave the ultimate religious authority to the Bishop of Rome, and made Roman Christianity the official religion of the state. He banned pagan sacrificial practices. During the fourth century, Christians grew from between five and seven percent of the population of the Roman Empire to fully half the empire's population. Mo'e conversions followed. None of this would have happened without the conversion of Constantine. It is difficult to envision any other sect of Christianity being attractive to the Roman emperor or providing such unifying effects on the empire. Becoming subject to Jewish Law, adopting a "new" religion like Marcion's, or an "elite" religion for the few who had "gnosis," would not have been attractive. If you could commune with God directly, through an inner "gnosis" you did not need a priest, let alone a bishop or pope to act as your intermediary or to tell you what to believe, or who to follow.

Constantine's conversion to the proto-Orthodox form of Christianity was undoubtedly the most important event in the subsequent rise of the Christian Church up until modern times. As a result, the victorious proto-Orthodox Christianity developed into the dominant religious, social, political and cultural institution of the West for centuries, and world's most populous religion.[40]

CHAPTER 5

What Did Jesus Really Say?

As mentioned in the Introduction, with the discovery of many new source documents in the Sinai Desert, and with the application of modern methods of textual analysis by scholars who are independent of institutional bias, most modern Biblical scholars will agree that the books of the Bible's New Testament are written at three levels of authenticity:

1. What were probably the actual words of Jesus, quoted in the Gospels of Matthew, Mark and Luke, but recorded several decades afterward.
2. What were probably interpolations, words attributed to Jesus by unknown sources.
3. What was said about Jesus or about his teachings by others, for example, Paul, in his "letters," which make up most of the rest of the New Testament, and which served as the basis for early Church dogma.

What do sayings at the first level reveal about who Jesus was and what his teachings were? Within Christianity and in the popular understanding of Jesus and his teaching, how much have sayings at the second and third levels distorted or obscured level number one? In this chapter, we present a discussion of those aphorisms, which the Jesus Seminar Fellows determined originated with Jesus himself. In doing so, the answers to the first question above will become especially apparent. The second and third questions will be answered primarily in the next chapter.

The aphorisms discussed below have been selected from the most authentic aphorisms attributed to Jesus by the Fellows of the Jesus Seminar, either undoubtedly (red) or probably (pink). These aphorisms are listed in Appendix A. They will also be compared to aphorisms from the writings of the Yoga Siddhas, to increase the understanding of their common source of inspiration.

Reversing Natural Human Inclinations

The scholars of the Jesus Seminar nominated a set of parodies as the most authentic verses in the New Testament.[1] A parody is an imitation of a style or form of discourse that exaggerates certain traits for comic effect. A case parody is the comic exaggeration of a law where certain features are overstated for effect. The following trio of case parodies was voted with a very high degree of consensus, as among the things Jesus almost certainly said:

"Don't react violently against the one who is evil; when someone slaps you on the right cheek, turn the other as well. When someone wants to sue you for your shirt, let that person have your coat along with it. Further, when anyone conscripts you for one mile, go an extra mile." (Matthew 5:39-41, with parallels in Luke 6.29)

"Give to the one who begs from you; and don't turn away the one who tries to borrow from you." (Matthew 5:42, with parallels in Luke 6.29)

"Love your enemies." (Matthew 5.43 with parallel in Luke 6:27-28)

Jesus asks us to do the opposite of what human nature would ordinarily cause us to do. Because the commands are so extreme, even ridiculous when taken literally (we'd all soon be naked and impoverished if we followed them to the limit), they give us the kind of insight that we could only have by becoming aware of the ordinary tendencies of the ego. They demand responses, which are just barely possible, so they enjoin us to go to the edge of human nature, and beyond. The admonition to "love your enemies" was ranked as the third highest among sayings that certainly originated with Jesus by the Fellows of the Jesus Seminar (after the clusters of aphorisms mentioned above). It is memorable because it cuts against the social grain and constitutes a paradox: those who love their enemies have no enemies.

This is also the method of Yoga and Tantra. As Sri Aurobindo put it humorously, when urged by his comrades who were fighting for India's independence from the British Empire to resume his political struggle, he quickly replied that what was needed was "not a revolt against the British Government, which anyone could easily manage…(but) a revolt against the whole of universal Nature."[2]

The "edge" of what the practitioner finds possible to do in a Yoga posture is the metaphor for the edges we reach in our human experience, for example, whenever we feel anger, fear or depression. By learning to keep our balance and our awareness, by keeping calm, listening, acting only after reflection, we extend what we are capable of doing, we stretch our human nature a little farther. Most of Yoga is doing the opposite of what our human nature would ordinarily cause us to do - remaining calm and content in the face of opposition or discord, sitting still, rather than moving, remaining awake when the eyes are closed, in meditation; allowing the breathing to slow to zero; being silent, rather than speaking; fasting rather than feasting; cultivating a witness consciousness instead of being absorbed in mental chatter.

"Be ye perfect, even as your Father in Heaven is perfect," (Matthew 5.48 with parallel in Luke 6:36). One of the meanings of the word for a yogic saint, Siddha is "one who has become perfect." Jesus challenged his listeners to perfect themselves, to overcome their lower human nature, and to become divine. Jesus, like the greatest of Yoga adepts, made his life his Yoga. He overcame all the ordinary limitations of the human existence to reveal his true nature, and more importantly, he admonished his listeners to do the same.

The Kingdom of Heaven

While scholars agree that Jesus spoke often about the "Kingdom of Heaven," or the "Kingdom of God," the question arises as to whether these phrases refer to God's direct intervention in the future, including the end of the world, and last judgment, or did Jesus use these terms to refer to something already present but elusive? The Fellows of the Jesus Seminar were inclined to believe that Jesus conceived the Kingdom of Heaven or God as being present all around but difficult to perceive. They did not believe that Jesus was referring to an apocalyptic vision, which was common among both earlier Jewish prophets and writers and later Church fathers, such as Paul and the author of Revelations. The confirming evidence of this conclusion lies in the major parables of Jesus: they do not reflect an apocalyptic view of history. Among his major parables were the good Samaritan, the prodigal son, the dinner party, the vineyard laborers, the shrewd manager, the unforgiving slave, the corrupt judge, the leaven in the flour, the mustard seed, the pearl of great price and the hidden treasure.

The parable of the mustard seed expressed his vision of the Kingdom of Heaven, and was voted by the Fellows as one of the parables most certainly spoken by Jesus.

"The followers said to Jesus, 'Tell us what heaven's kingdom is like.' He said to them, 'It is like a mustard seed. (It) is the smallest of all seeds, but when it falls on prepared soil, it produces a large plant and becomes a shelter for birds of heaven.'" (Gospel of Thomas Saying 20, with parallel verses in Mark 4.30-32, Luke 13.18-19, and Matthew 13. 31-32)

The metaphor of the mustard seed (proverbial for its smallness) is considered by scholars to be a good example of how Jesus considered God's domain to be: modest, common and pervasive, rather than imperial. They point out that the mighty cedar of Lebanon tree (Ezekial 17:22-23) and the apocalyptic tree of Daniel (Daniel 4:12, 20-22) were the traditional metaphors used to describe God's domain. Jesus' selection of the mustard tree pokes fun at established tradition in a comical way. It is also anti-social in that it endorses counter movements and ridicules established tradition. The version in Thomas is considered to be closest to the original, as the versions of this in the Synoptic Gospels describe the mustard plant as a tree or biggest of all garden plants, thus accommodating the apocalyptic tree theme of the Hebrew scriptures, and misinterpreting the original message of Jesus.[3]

The parable of the leaven in the flour also teaches us about the Kingdom of Heaven, and how reversing our human nature permits us to perceive it.

"The Kingdom of Heaven is like leaven which a woman took and concealed in fifty pounds of flour until it was all leavened." (Matthew 13.33, parallels in Luke 13.20-21 and Thomas 96)

This one-sentence parable transmits the voice of Jesus as clearly as any ancient record can, in the judgment of the Fellows of the Jesus Seminar. He uses three images in a way that would have been very surprising to His audience. "Hiding" leaven in flour is an unusual way to express the idea of mixing yeast and flour. It implies that God has deliberately concealed His Kingdom from us. The surprise increases when Jesus notes that there were "fifty pounds" of flour. In Genesis 18, three men, representatives of God, appear to Abraham and promise him and his wife that she will conceive a child soon, even though she is aged. For the occasion, Sarah is instructed to make cakes of fifty pounds of flour to give to the heavenly visitors. Fifty pounds of flour must be a suitable quantity to celebrate an epiphany (Greek – "the appearance; miraculous phenomenon"), a visible, though indirect manifestation of God. The third image is the use of leaven, regarded as a symbol of corruption by the Judeans. In the Passover celebration, bread was made without leaven. In a surprising reversal of the customary associations, the leaven here represents not what is corrupt and unholy, but the Kingdom of God. This is a typical strategy of Jesus, according to the Fellows of the Jesus Seminar.[4] That God deliberately hides his Kingdom from us is one of the "five functions of the Lord," namely obscuration, according to Saiva Siddhanta (see below). It obliges us to seek Him, to overcome the delusion of the world.

"In His Grace was I born;

In His Grace I grew up;

In His Grace I rested in death;

In His Grace I was in obfuscation;

In His Grace I tasted of ambrosial bliss;

In His Grace, *Nandi* (the Lord) entered."

(*Thirumandiram*, verse 1800)

Thomas 113 tells us that the Kingdom of Heaven is already here, but that we do not see it:

His disciples said to him, "When will the (Father's) imperial rule come?" "It will not come by watching for it. It will not be said, "Look, here!" or "Look, there!" Rather, the Father's imperial rule is spread out upon the earth, and people don't see it."[5]

Jesus' contemporary, the Yoga Siddha Thirumular affirms this same truth, that God's Kingdom is here, but that ordinary people do not see it:

"They who do not see the Treasure that surpasses all,

But seek the treasures that perish,

If within their melting heart they seek inside

They will see the Treasure that dies not."

-*Thirumandiram*, verse 762

On Entering into the Kingdom of Heaven

"For it is easier for a camel to go through a needle's eye, than for a rich man to enter into the kingdom of God." (Mark 10.25, with parallels in Matthew 19.24 and Luke 18.25)

This aphorism is graphic and humorous and exhibits Jesus' use of hyperbole and exaggeration. "It cannot be taken literally, which suggests that the whole discussion of the relation of wealth to God's Kingdom should be viewed circumspectly: does Jesus literally mean that everyone should embrace poverty as a way of life? Poverty and celibacy are aspects of the ascetic life that became popular in the Christian movement at an early date. The Fellows of the Jesus Seminar believe that these impulses did not stem from Jesus."[6]

This aphorism is also part of a complex of aphorisms, which describe how difficult it is for those with money to enter God's kingdom. The more material things one has, the greater the risk of becoming attached to them, and consequently missing "the Kingdom of Heaven." Jesus had blessed the poor in the beatitudes, telling them that God's domain belonged to them, so he probably believed that in simplicity, one was closer to the living Presence of the Lord. It reflects the view that attachment to material things prevents one from realizing the spiritual dimension.[7] It is not the material things themselves that are problematic, but the desire and attachments for them, which keeps us in ignorance and causes us to lose sight of the Reality of God's Kingdom all around us. It is the deluding tendency of the mind to fantasize, worry and become preoccupied with things, absorbed in them, rather than to live freely, identified as self-effulgent awareness, "in the light." He is also encouraging his listeners to go beyond the duality of poor-rich, hungry-not hungry, weeping-comforted, in other words the disease of the mind, in which one ordinarily identifies with one body, mind and emotions. One must purify oneself of desires, in order to transcend the ego's perspective that "I am the body" and its attachment to the body's pleasures.

> "Blessed are the poor, for theirs is the kingdom of heaven,
>
> Blessed are the hungry, for you will feast,
>
> Blessed are those who weep, for you will be comforted."
>
> (Luke 6.21, with parallels in Thomas 54, 69.2, 58 and Matthew 5.3, 5.6)

Analysis of the collection of sayings known as the beatitudes by scholars has revealed that the above three were almost certainly spoken by Jesus, but that they circulated separately in the oral tradition. The scholars found no "Sermon on the Mount" in which he spoke to a large crowd the collection of beatitudes. In fact it was the oral repetition under different circumstances and on different occasions, which led to individual variations in their recording in the Gospels. Four of them were eventually combined into one series by the author of Q, probably on the basis of common form. Matthew and Luke took over the complex and modified and expanded it.

"Blessed are you when people hate you, when they persecute you, and denounce you and scorn your name as evil, because of the son of man." (Luke 6.22-23, with parallels in Matthew 5.10-12, Thomas 68.1-2, 69.1)

This fourth beatitude may go back to Jesus in some earlier form, in which it had to do with those who suffer now. In its present form, however, it reflects conditions of the Christian community after persecution had set in.

Saying that the poor are blessed, or in modern terms, "congratulating the poor without qualification is unexpected, to say the least, and even paradoxical, since congratulations were normally extended only to those who enjoyed prosperity, happiness, or power. The congratulations addressed to the weeping and the hungry are expressed in vivid and exaggerated language, which announces a dramatic transformation."[8]

(Matthew's version added another four beatitudes, which offer reward for virtue rather than relief from distress. There is no surprise, no reversal, no paradox, as was characteristic of the sayings of Jesus.)

The irony and paradox employed in these beatitudes also reminds us of the manner of teaching of the Yoga Siddhas. These teachings help us come to understand that regardless of what appears to be going on in our life, the only place anything is really happening is in our mind. Each of us is blessed as "the son of man," regardless of what mental reaction and mental limitation we are experiencing at the moment. For our true being is seated beyond the senses that take in, and react to what is happening about us; it is beyond the conditioning of the mind and the intellect, which interprets what is being seen, head, tasted, touch and felt. Our true being and nature is blessed, seated secretly in limitless, illuminated bliss. With this understanding we can transcend the ordinary human consciousness, the perspective of the ego, and access the perspective of our soul, which is one of peace and unconditional joy, in short, beatitude.

In the *Yoga-Sutras*, Patanjali tells us that "By austerity, impurities of the body and senses are destroyed and perfection gained." *Yoga-sutra* II.43[9] Classical *Yoga*, as expounded by Patanjali tells us that we are dreaming with our eyes open, because we identify not with what we are, which is pure consciousness, but with what we are not, our dreams, the movements of the mind. This apparent and mistaken identification of the Self or Seer, with the manifestations of nature (the Seen) is the fundamental cause of human suffering and the fundamental problem of human consciousness. The Self is the pure, absolute subject, and is experienced as "I am." But in ordinary human consciousness, the Self has become an object: "myself", a personality, an ego ridden collection of thoughts, feelings and sensations which assumes the role of the subject. The habit of identifying with our thoughts, emotions, sensations, that is, egoism is the nearly universal disease of ordinary human consciousness. It is only by ceasing to identify with these, through the process of detachment and purification, that one can realize one's true identity: the Self. The Self and the Lord have one common element, consciousness, according to Patanjali and the Siddhas, and it is by the realization of our true Self, that we can also realize the Lord, and be in His Kingdom.[10]

Why Should Jesus Say that Those Who are Poor, Hungry, Suffering and Persecuted are Blessed?

This is a great religious blessing and also instructive to help common man hold onto the basic principles of living life in the world, even when he suffers at the hands of the world.

Yoga Siddhas would say that the pure witness consciousness of the soul does not emerge in the world full grown, strong and luminous, it must evolve from its first stunted and feeble state. It must evolve by passing through various trials and sufferings. The soul is mired in the ignorance and unconsciousness of the worldly manifestation. The soul must emerge from Nature unscathed by suffering or persecution. It must become more and more perfect in order that it can impress upon what it receives upon its outer instrument, the body, mind and emotions. In addition, we are reminded that unless the outer instrument suffers, it will not seek or receive the soul's attention.

The beatitudes (Latin – "perfect happiness") are paradoxical statements, which call for a deep reflection upon their meaning. Given Jesus' repeated assertions that the Kingdom of God is already present, the beatitudes are not a promise of a future reward in some heavenly afterlife, as is usually interpreted by those who believe Jesus was announcing the end of the world. Are they not, rather, a challenge to his listeners to transform their condition into a means of purification? It is a direct challenge to let go of the feeling, "I am suffering," "I am poor," "I am hungry," and to realize that "I am not the body," "I am not my emotions," "I am not my suffering" and "I am not my mind." "I am" is closer to the Truth. It is a challenge to be the Witness of your life, to be the Seer, not the Seen.

Yoga teaches that the life ordinarily brings with it much suffering. This is because of ignorance of our true divine identity. Patanjali tells us in *Yoga-sutra* II.3, the causes of suffering: "Ignorance, egoism, attachment, aversion and clinging to life are the five afflictions." When we suffer, we begin to question, and we seek wisdom to answer the fundamental questions of life: "Who am I?" "Where did I come from?" "Why am I here?" "Why am I suffering?" We need the light of wisdom to see beyond our suffering. Wisdom is what dispels ignorance. Patanjali tells us that "Ignorance is seeing the impermanent as permanent, the impure as pure, the painful as pleasurable and the non-Self as the Self."[11] As we begin to realize wisdom and dispel ignorance, we can begin to see the grace of the Lord acting through our suffering, helping us to turn towards Him. If we apply the lessons of wisdom of Jesus, we can find our way back to the Lord in this life. We need not wait for heaven; we can begin to experience the joy of the Lord in every moment of every day. This is what the mystics discover.

On Purity

"Listen to me, all of you, and try to understand! It's not what goes into a person from the outside that can defile; rather it's what comes out of the person that defiles." (Mark 7.14-15 with parallels in Matthew 15.10-11 and Thomas 14.5)

"This aphorism is a categorical challenge to the laws governing pollution and purity. Since the saying need not be taken entirely literally – although it certainly has a literal dimension with respect to foods – it can also be made to apply to other forms of pollution, as Mark explained. It is characteristic of Jesus: it challenges the everyday, the inherited, the established, and erases social boundaries taken to be sacrosanct. If Jesus taught that there is nothing taken into the mouth that can defile, he was undermining a whole way of life."[12]

As a means of entering the Kingdom of God through purification, Jesus insists here on the true purity: inner purity, as distinct from the external rules emphasized by the Pharisees. Inner purity, of the heart, begins with discrimination against thoughts, words and actions that defile: judgment, greed, lust, anger, hatred, desire. All of them cause suffering for others and for the person harboring them. Words and actions are preceded by thoughts, so one must develop awareness of the negative mental tendencies and detach from them as soon as they begin to manifest within us.

The Siddhas, like Patanjali take a direct approach to such negative thoughts and tendencies: "When bound by negative thoughts, their opposite should be cultivated." (*Yoga-sutra* II.33)[13] But Patanjali's main yogic method was the cultivation of detachment towards them, letting go of identifying with the mental movements. The purifying process of Classical Yoga can be summarized in two acts of spiritual discipline: "Yoga is remembering Who Am I, and letting go of what I am not." Like the two wings of a bird, they lift one to Heaven. This reminds one of the new Christian motto: "What would Jesus do?"

On Worry, and Being Present

"That's why I tell you: Don't fret about your life – what you are going to eat and drink – or about your body – what you are going to wear. There is more to living than food and clothing, isn't there? Take a look at the birds of the sky: they don't plant or harvest, or gather into barns. Yet your heavenly Father feeds them. You are worth more than they, aren't you? Can any of you add one hour to life by fretting about it? Why worry about clothes? Notice how the wild lilies grow: they don't slave and they never spin. Yet let me tell you, even Solomon at the height of his glory was never decked out like one of them. If God dresses up the grass in the field, which is here today and tomorrow is thrown into an oven, won't (God care) for you even more, you who don't take anything for granted? So, don't fret. Don't say, "What am I going to eat?" or "What am I going to drink" or "What am I going to wear?"" (Matthew 6.25-31, with parallels in Luke 12.22-31 and Thomas 36)

This is one of the most important things that Jesus said. It is also, according to the scholars of the Jesus Seminar, probably the longest connected discourse that can be directly attributed to Jesus (with the exception of some of the longer narrative parables). Most of it comes from Q. This string of sayings was addressed to those who are preoccupied with day-to-day survival, rather than with political or apocalyptic crises. Jesus believed that God would provide for human needs. They are also connected with his saying, "Blessed are the hungry," (Luke 6.21) petition for the day's bread (Mathew 6.11) and the certainty that those who ask will receive. (Luke 11:10) Drawing upon figures of speech from the everyday world, these figures challenge the common attitudes towards life. They are exaggerations: humans are not fed like birds and are not clothed like the grass of the field.[14]

By encouraging his listeners to live in the present, Jesus was reminding them that it is only here, now, where they can find the Kingdom of God. By letting go of worries, and appreciating the present moment, one can develop the mystic vision of the Absolute Intelligence at work in the Universe. One can see how the God through Nature provides us with what we need to grow and evolve into His Own Image.

This echoes Patanjali's famous aphorisms: "Yoga is the cessation of identifying with the fluctuations arising within consciousness. The Seer abides in his own true form."[15] In the ordinary human mind, worries obscure the vision, so one fails to see the ever-present Being. All spiritual traditions, including Yoga and that to which Jesus belonged, taught the value of cultivating mental silence and equanimity. In doing so, we purify ourselves of the false identities of the ego.

On Aspiration

"Ask, and it shall be given you; seek, and you will find; knock, and it will be opened for you. Rest assured: everyone who asks receives; everyone who seeks finds; and for the one who knocks it is opened. Who among you would hand a son a stone when it is bread he's asking for? Again, who would hand him a snake when it is fish he's asking for? Of course no one would! So if you, shiftless as you are, know how to give your children good gifts, isn't it much more likely that your Father in the heavens will give good things to those who ask him?" (Matthew 7.7-11)[16]

Here, Jesus is not referring to the ordinary prayers, which are generally petitions for things which our ego believes that it needs to be happy. Rather he is addressing what is referred to in yogic literature as "aspiration," for Self knowledge. Sri Aurobindo defines aspiration as "a spiritual enthusiasm, the height and ardor of the soul's seeking."[17] Aspiration is the call of the soul for the Lord Himself. Desire is the cry of the ego, for something it imagines that it needs to be happy. Aspiration is the opposite of desire. One is intensely aware of the limitations of the ego-bound existence, and one seeks to come out of its prison. One directs one's energies away from the ego-center. It first manifests as a thirst for spiritual knowledge, and later as a quiet, steady seeking of the Divine Itself. It is a spiritual enthusiasm of our soul towards perfection, unconditional love, truth and beauty. Grace is the response of the Lord to the soul's call. It reflects the widespread recognition that prayers are answered by a source of benevolence, independent of whether we are deserving or not. With grace, we receive what is uplifting and edifying for our soul, in response to its call.

Aspiration in the practice of Yoga, may take the form of intensive austerities, known as *tapas*, with the purpose of surrendering one ego, and its desires and fears, to the Lord. And when this is done in a sacred way, for a prolonged period, the intense spiritual energy within and without facilitates spiritual experiences and much grace. From late 1972 to early 1973, I performed 48 days of prayer and yogic practices *(tapas)* at the Brahmanoor Kali temple in a small village in Kanadukathan, Tamil Nadu, India. Every night at midnight I went there, made a small ceremony, and then sat in deep meditation for several hours. The very small temple consisted of a large stone slab, with a corrugated tin roof, and mud brick walls. About fifty years earlier, this "temple" was constructed by an American railway engineer, who was supervising the construction of the railway line running less than fifty yards behind the present temple. In a dream one night an Indian goddess appeared to him, and told him to divert the railway line, away from a certain spot, and to dig up an image of her that was buried there. As soon as he awoke, he began to direct some of his construction crew to dig in the place about which he had dreamed. There they found the image of Mother Goddess. The image was a large round stone, with a carved head on it. It resembled a stone-age earth mother carving more than anything. He was so moved by the experience that he had a small temple built there in honor of the Divine Mother. In 1948, a terrible drought affected this region. There was no rain for more than three years. A famous Yoga Siddha, Prasananda Guru was summoned. He performed non-stop yogic *tapas* at this temple for 48 days. On the forty eighth day it rained, and since that time, there have been no droughts. Prasananda Guru became one of the first teachers of my teacher, Yogi Ramaiah.

The temple was located in a barren, desert like area. Although lacking in adornments, it had an intense spiritual energy. At night, many cobras came out of their holes and circulated around it. Surrendering my fear, in the darkness, engulfed in the temple's intense spiritual energy, my meditations became extraordinarily deep, and I often entered the breathless state of meditation, known as *samadhi*. The effects of these nocturnal sessions carried over during the day. Even as I went through my day I remained in a state of witnessing transcendence in which "I" experienced myself one with everything. I was so deeply content. God was everywhere.

Tapas means literally, "to heat," or "straightening by fire," and it can be used as a voluntary self-challenge to overcome anything in one's nature, or as a penance to atone for past misdeeds, but in Yoga it is used primarily to cultivate the fire of aspiration: to surrender the ego's perspective and to realize God.

Yogis would recognize the forty days Jesus spent in the wilderness as Yogic *tapas*. His great aspiration to surrender all desires, all temptations, to want only the Father, were all characteristic of what advanced Yogis do to purify themselves, and enter into a state of communion with the Lord.

Showing the Path to Others

"Since when is the lamp brought in to be put under the bushel basket or under the bed? It is put on the lamp stand, isn't it? After all there is nothing hidden except to be brought to the light, nor anything secreted away that won't be exposed." (Mark 4.21-22 with parallels in Luke 8.16; Matt. 5.15, Luke 11:33 and Thomas 33.2-3)

The same saying appears in three different sources, Mark, Thomas, and Q, and in five different times in the Gospels, in slightly different contexts. This fact illustrates the rule of evidence that Jesus' followers remembered only the gist of his sayings rather than his precise words. The different contexts demonstrate as well that the Evangelists often make up contexts for the sayings of Jesus.

"The motif of the aphorism is light; it is connected with other sayings in which light, or sight, or disclosure is a motif. The point being made is that the light is not meant to be hidden. In Matthew, it is because the disciples are the community of the beatitudes (5.3-12) that they are the light of the world. In Mark 4.21 and Luke 8.16, it is because the disciples have been given sight: they see the meaning of the parables and should share their insight with others. Luke has grouped this saying with others about the light that illuminates the body (11:33-36). In Thomas 33.2-3, it is the hidden truth coming to "light" through the ear."[18] In all of these contexts, "light" is a metaphor for higher consciousness or insight.

This is similar to the concept of *arrupadai* ("showing the path to others") in the Siddha literature. This is expressed in Thirumular's famous aphorism: "May this world share the bliss that I have had." The social concern of the Siddhas included not only their physical well being, but sharing the wisdom and means to removing the sources of suffering.

The following verse from the Siddha Boganathar illustrates not only his concern of showing others where to find the "light" but also where not to find it: in doubtful religions practices and penances:

"Abandon the doubtful twelve religions;

Withdraw from the possessive religious worship and meditations;

All is illusory; the result is nothing.

Three are the *nadis* (energy channels) of the lustrous *kundalini* ("coiling like a snake;" "serpent power"),

Encircling and enclosing the *manipura* (*chakra*) in the middle of the abdomen;

It stands united with the magnificent Supreme Being.

I am unable to see anything other than you (who is) forever permanent."

- Astanga Yoga 24, verse 13[19]

The simplest form of this aphorism of Jesus appears in Thomas 5.2, where it consists of a single line: "There is nothing hidden that will not be revealed." In the context of parable interpretation, this saying can only mean that the secrets of the parables are intended to be revealed. If so, it is puzzling why those secrets were hidden in the first place. The answer the Evangelists give to that question is so "they (the outsiders) may look but not see, listen but not understand."[20]

The appended aphorism about the need for the hidden to be brought to light and the explanation of why everything is in parables appears to be contradictory. The confusion undoubtedly is due to the attempt of early interpreters to reconcile two opposing themes in the Jesus tradition: (1)

Jesus taught in parables that were difficult to understand; and (2) Jesus insisted that his teachings were meant to shed light, to be understood, to be revealing. In imitation of Mark, Luke attempts to utilize these appended proverbs to explain this paradox.

This is similar to the deliberately obscure twilight language used by the Siddhas in their poetry. Is it so puzzling why these secrets are hidden or obscured in the first place? The language is intended to hide certain truths from those who are not yet ready to know the absolute truth. Who is really ready to experience God?

The language of the Siddhas and of Jesus contains several layers of meaning, both at the level of ordinary experience and of transcendence. It is both suggestive and paradoxical. The language itself is mystical in nature, where the highest is clothed in the form of the lowest. The Siddhas made free use of typology, wordplay, paradox, repetition, and metaphor to convey to the listener the richness of the reality hidden in the visible terms and symbols. The true meaning of the expression is accessible only to the initiated. It is likely that the Siddha poems themselves functioned as an initiation. It is a language for preaching esoteric, mystical doctrines.[21]

The saying of Jesus: "When thine eye is single, thy whole body shall be full of light," (Luke 11.34) refers to mystical teachings given by Jesus to his most worthy disciples, during secret initiations. Students of Kundalini Yoga would recognize it as referring to the opening of the *ajna chakra*, or third eye, between the eyebrows. The light of higher, consciousness comes to those who open this *ajna chakra* according to the Siddha literature.

The message of not hiding our light is not as straightforward as one might think. When to show it? How? To who? Who is ready to see it? In 1976, during a cross country pilgrimage with Yogi Ramaiah, I was given a memorable example of this problem. We stopped one night to camp near Pike's Peak. Yogi Ramaiah told us that he was going to go into the forest to do *sadhana* (meditation) alone, but that no one should follow him. This last statement greatly aroused my curiosity, and after much internal debate, I decided to follow him, keeping very quiet so as not to create any disturbance. Deep in the forest he sat down against a tree and entered a state of meditation. I hid behind another tree, about fifty feet away. His eyes were open; however they were turned up completely, revealing only the whites of his eyes, indicating a deep state. Then, to my surprise his body began to glow. The glow became so great that I could no longer distinguish his human form. There was only a ball of light where I had perceived his physical form. I rubbed my eyes and pinched myself to convince myself that I was not dreaming. The ball of light persisted for over thirty minutes. I was filled with joy perceiving it. Gradually the light grew dimmer, and I could again perceive his familiar form. His eyes closed, and then opened again and got up and began to walk back towards our camp. Then, out of the corner of his eye, he spotted me crouching behind a tree. He gently scolded me, saying: "I said that no one should follow me."

Later, I asked him what he was doing, by stopping at various places and going into such states. He replied that he was "planting seeds;" that the spiritual energy, which he was leaving at each place would eventually stimulate the spiritual development of people in America. He remarked that the American Indians had left many such spiritual seeds, in special places, and that these would also bear fruit one day.

The Lord's Prayer

The prayer as it probably appeared in the Gospel Q:

Abba (Father)

Your name be revered

Impose your imperial come (Thy Kingdom come)

Provide us with the bread we need for the day

Forgive our debts to the extent we have forgiven those in debt to us

And please don't subject us to test after test.[22]

The Fellows of the Jesus Seminar agreed that where Luke 11:2-4 and Matt 6.9-13 exactly agree, they are reproducing the Q text. It is unlikely, in the judgment of the Fellows, that Jesus taught his disciples the prayer as a whole, even in its reconstructed form. They think it is more likely, given the conditions under which oral discourse is transmitted, that he employed the four petitions from time to time but as individual prayers. He of course, frequently used *Abba* to address God. Someone in the Q community probably assembled the prayer for the first time; Matthew and Luke then copied the Q version, while editing and revising it at the same time.

Abba is the Aramaic word for Father. Scholars agree that Jesus referred to God with this name. In Judea, the name for God was sacred and it was forbidden to utter it aloud. Among the Jewish Essenes, a person was expelled from the community for pronouncing the name of God, even accidentally. Yet Jesus used a familiar form of address and then asked that the name be regarded as sacred – a paradox that seems characteristic of Jesus' teachings.[23]

The word for Father in the Tamil language used by the Siddhas of south India was *Appa*. There is no letter "b" in Tamil, so the Siddhas referred to the Lord with the same familiar term as Jesus did. Why this is so is not evident.

God's Unconditional Love

The parable of the prodigal son (Luke 15. 11-32) is ranked among the two dozen or so sayings in the gospels, which were probably spoken by Jesus. It is the longest, and its message of God's unconditional love for all souls is, along with the presence of the Kingdom of God, the most important.

"Once there was this man who had two sons. The younger of them said to his father, 'Father, give me the share of my property that's coming to me.' So he divided his resources between them.

Not too many days later, the younger son got all his things together and left home for a faraway country, where he squandered property by living extravagantly. Just when he had spent it all, a serious famine swept through that country, and he began to do without. So he went and hired himself out to one of the citizens of that country, who sent him out to his farm to feed the pigs. He longed to satisfy his hunger with the carob pods, which the pigs usually ate; but no one offered him anything. Coming to his senses he said, "Lots of my father's hired hands have more than enough to eat, while here I am dying of starvation! I'll get up and go to my father and I'll say to him 'Father, I have sinned against heaven and affronted you; I don't deserve to be called a son of yours any longer; treat me like one of your hired hands.' And he got up and returned to his father.

But the father said to his slaves, 'Quick! Bring out the finest robe and put it on him; put a ring on his finger and sandals on his feet. Fetch the fat calf and slaughter it; let's have a feast and celebrate, because this son of mine was dead and has come back to life; he was lost and now is found.' And they started celebrating.

Now his elder son was out in the field; and as he got closer to the house, heard music and dancing. He called one of the servant-boys over and asked what was going on.

He said to him, 'Your brother has come home and your father has slaughtered the fat calf, because he has him back safe and sound.'

But he was angry and refused to go in. So his father came out and began to plead with him. But he answered his father, 'See here, all these years I have slaved for you. I never once disobeyed any of your orders; yet you never once provided me with a kid goat so I could celebrate with my friends. But when this son of yours shows up, the one who has squandered your estate with prostitutes – for him you slaughter the fat calf.'

But (the father) said to him, 'My child, you are always at my side. Everything that's mine is yours. But we just had to celebrate and rejoice, because this brother of yours was dead, and has come back to life; he was lost and now is found.'"[24]

Jesus' parable was primarily intended as a lesson of forgiveness and unconditional love. Its lesson is that those who have always remained with God should forgive those who have truly repented and returned and should receive them with love, rejoicing in their return.

Christian teaching identifies Jesus with the father, in this parable, but in a parable, like a dream or poem, the teller is all the images and characters. I include Stephen Mitchell's insightful commentary on this aspect of this wonderful parable: "...any separation from God is painful to a young man of Jesus' gifts, and the smallest mistake appears huge under the microscope of his moral conscience. Not even the greatest Masters were spared the process of spiritual death and rebirth. For Jesus, the rebirth must have been particularly astonishing because it had to include and overcome the sustained indignities of his childhood... I don't want to suggest that Jesus be identified only with the younger son. It is also true that he is the father, that wonderful figure whose delicate, loving treatment of the older son calls for as much admiration as his unconditional acceptance of the younger son. And he is also the older son, whose grievances are stated harshly but fairly, and whom the parable treats with the tolerance and respect so disastrously lacking in the inauthentic Gospel sayings about the righteous. But if we look for the parable's center of gravity, we can recognize that Jesus is the younger son at least as much as he is the father. And when the son returns to the father, all his shame and sorrow and unworthiness are taken up into the father's uncontainable joy. At this point, the story steps out of the son's consciousness into the father's; in a sense, the son becomes the father. There is no longer any difference between the exhilaration of being forgiven and the joy of forgiving."[25]

This is a particularly powerful parable, which expresses the need to continue to progress towards the Lord. To continue the process of creating and recreating ourselves in His Image until we abide in the qualities of the Lord. We are throughout existence in a constant mutable rhythm of movement. Either we are moving outward from God or we are being brought closer to Him, moved by pleasure, pain and neutral indifference. Most movements away and toward are discordant as they are the tangled responses arising from an imperfect and not yet fully conscious being. Both the older and the younger brother are in this state of moving toward and away from that perfect center- a conscious state of Being.

God's forgiveness and unconditional love is also central to the teaching of the Siddhas. The Siddhas taught that God's Love and Force carries us through all the stages of our lives, all our suffering, ups and downs and in all His Divine functions. Why? The *Saiva Siddhanta*, philosophy of South Indian Siddhas explains it thus: The Lord, known as *pati* (literally, "Lord"), the *pasu* (individual soul), and the *pasas*, (bonds of egoism, *karma* (cause and effect) and maya (manifestation of world appearance) are the three eternal realities. The Lord has five functions: creation, preservation, destruction, obscuration and grace. These are His alone, and they distinguish Him from God-realized souls. Through the Lord, souls gain the experience they need to find their way back to Godhead. In *Tirumandiram* verse 2418, Tirumular, a contemporary of Jesus, said, "Creation, Preservation, and Dissolution, (That for the souls grant rest from the whirl of birth-and-death) Obfuscation and Grace (That redeem souls, after life below). What is the Lord's purpose in performing His several activities?" "It is just His play." Play does not mean amusement. It means that it is out of the sheer bliss of creating and recreating Himself in Himself, the Lord performs His activities, for self-creation and self- representation. He Himself is the play; He Himself is the player; He Himself is the playground. God performs all these actions with ease, without undergoing any change. He does this out of love of the souls. It is His grace that actuates His activities. The reason is to help the souls to be rid of their fetters or *pasa* (their bondage to the world).[26] Jesus' parable of the prodigal son reflects this purpose: both sons loses their way in the delusion of the world. It takes remembering whose son they are, and why they are here to become freed from their delusion. The younger son experiences complete liberation from his suffering due to the unconditional love of his father. The elder son is taught to remember whose son he is, and brought to understand the true reason for living a life in the world.

The following verse clearly states this:

"It was His grace that led me into *pasa*

> It was His grace that freed me from that *pasa*
>
> It was His grace that in divine love granted *mukti* (liberation from Nature)
>
> It was His grace that granted me the love
>
> For the state beyond *mukti*"
>
> (*Tirumandiram* 1802)

How can it be said that these are acts of grace when most of these other acts of the Lord plunge the souls into birth and death and thus make them suffer? The *Tirumandiram* answers:

> "In His Grace I was born
>
> In His Grace I grew up
>
> In His Grace I rested in death;
>
> In His Grace I was in obfuscation;
>
> In His Grace I tasted of ambrosial bliss;
>
> In His Grace, *Nandi (*the Lord*)*, my heart entered."
>
> (*Tirumandiram* 1800)

"That is, the act of "creation" is carried out by Him to enable the souls by giving them a body, etc., to work out their respective karmas; "sustenance" is to make the souls experience the fruit of their action; "destruction" is to give rest to the souls; "obfuscation" is to veil the nature of souls as consciousness and bring about indifference to fruits of their good and bad actions, by first making them engage in action; "grace" is the grant of release. All these activities are thus indicative of His Grace."[27]

Forgiveness of Sins and the Karmic Consequences of our Actions

Closely related to the theme of Jesus' teaching of unconditional love is the forgiveness of sins. The parable of the shrewd manager (Luke 16.1-8) illustrates this:

"There was this rich man whose manager had been accused of squandering his master's property. He called him in and said, 'What's this I hear about you? Let's have an audit of your management, because your job is being terminated.'

Then the manager said to himself, 'What am I going to do? My master is firing me. I'm not strong enough to dig ditches and I'm ashamed to beg. I've got it! I know what I'll do so doors will open for me when I'm removed from management.'

So he called in each of his master's debtors. He said to the first, 'How much do you owe my master?'

He said, 'Five hundred gallons of olive oil.'

And he said to him, 'Here is your invoice; sit down right now and make it two hundred and fifty.'

Then he said to another, "And how much do you owe?"

He said, 'A thousand bushels of wheat.'

He says to him, 'Here is your invoice; make it eight hundred.'

'The master praised the dishonest manager because he had acted shrewdly.'"

This parable troubled its earliest Christian interpreters. The several sayings Luke has attached to it are attempts to moralize and soften it. (Luke 16.8b-13) Some fellows of the Jesus Seminar consider "the master praised the dishonest manager because he had acted shrewdly" to be an appended conclusion, not integral to the parable and not customary in Jesus' parables. But most fellows regarded it to be a part of the parable, as it provided a surprising twist that is characteristic of Jesus' metaphorical stories. This story does not moralize, nor does it commend crooked dealing or accounting.[28] Then what is its message?

The dishonest manager was forgiven by his master because he forgave, in part, the debts of others. Similarly, God forgives us when we forgive others. It echoes what was included in the Lord's Prayer, discussed above: "Forgive our debts to the extent we have forgiven those in debt to us." It is also consistent with the teaching of unconditional love in the parable of the prodigal son.

The Old Testament prophets and their followers, the Pharisees, emphasized a legal conception of our relationship with God. God makes laws. If you transgress those laws, God will judge and punish you. Jesus brought a new message: God loves you. And your sins against the law are forgiven when you recognize them and make amends. Rather than fearing Him, learn to love Him. He is at hand.

In this parable, notice that everyone was held to account, and were still required to pay the greater part of their debt. This reflects the metaphysical teaching about karma, that all actions, words and thoughts have consequences, but that there is a higher metaphysical law, that of grace, which can mitigate the consequences of karma, when we seek the Lord Himself. Bad karma, that which causes suffering, can be countered with good karma, that which forgives others for their transgressions against us or brings joy to others. Unlike karma, however, Grace is bestowed when we seek the Lord. This is consistent with the teachings of Jesus that the Kingdom of God is at hand, and that if we seek him, we will find him and his blessings. The parable teaches us that all of us are prone to make mistakes, but when we recognize that the consequences are always there, and that God loves us despite our errors, we are freed from our fear of the Lord, and learn to love him without conditions, as He loves us.

The Siddha Tirumular's famous saying drives home the point that God (Siva) is love, and that when we truly realize what love is, we also realize God (Siva):

> "The ignorant prate that Love and Siva are two,
>
> But none do know that Love alone is Siva
>
> When men but know that Love and Siva are the same,
>
> Love as Siva, they ever remained."

(*Tirumandiram*, verse 270)

Hidden Treasure

There is not an unbridgeable gulf between God and man. The parables of Jesus and the Siddhas create a bridge between them. The tendency of the ordinary mind, to discredit, to make divisions, and to distinguish this from that, makes very difficult the discernment of Oneness, the truth behind all that exists. The power of these parables is that they contain hidden treasures. They contain a pregnant vibration, which has the power to continue to evolve itself, within the consciousness of the individual reading them.

The parable of hidden treasure is comparable to the behavior of the shrewd manager who swindles his master in order to provide for his own future.

"Heaven's imperial rule ("the Kingdom of Heaven" in the King James version) is like a treasure in a field: when someone finds it, that person covers it up again, and out of sheer joy goes and sells every last possession and buys that field.

Again, Heaven's imperial rule is like some trader looking for beautiful pearls. When that merchant finds one priceless pearl, he sells everything he owns and buys it." (Matthew 13.44-46, Thomas 109: 1-3, and Thomas 76: 1-2)[29]

Surprising stories like this, in which Jesus employs a dubious moral example, are characteristic of Jesus' parable technique. In these two parables, he is in effect saying that loving God and finding his Kingdom are more important than conventional morality. Love surpasses the limitations of the Law. He uses shocking, extreme examples to shake his listeners out of their fear of God, and their blind obedience to the numerous laws that governed Judaism.

The Siddha Tirumular also points to the whereabouts of the "hidden treasure," God Himself within:

"The Lord God know them who, by night and day,

Seat Him in heart's core, and in love exalted adore;

To them wise with inner light, action less in trance,

He comes, and, in close proximity, stands before."

(*Tirumandiram*, verse 288)

The Good Samaritan

In Luke 10.30-35 Jesus tells the story: There was a man traveling from Jerusalem down to Jericho when he fell victim to robbers. He was stripped, beaten, and left half dead. Within a short time, a priest traveling that same road caught sight of the injured man; yet, the priest went out of his way to avoid him. Similarly, when a Levite came upon the man, he took one look and crossed the road in avoidance. But, then came a Samaritan, who coming upon the man was moved in empathy. He went straight to his aid, caring for his wounds, pouring olive oil and wine on them. He hoisted him onto his own animal, brought him to an inn, and looked after him. The next day he took from his own pocket two silver coins, giving them to the innkeeper, he said, "Look after him, and on my way back I'll reimburse you for any extra expense you have had."

Luke's narrative is closely integrated with its context. Jesus and the legal expert engage in a dialogue in which the question is raised: "Who is my neighbor?" (Luke 10.25-29) The parable furnishes Luke with an answer and his readers with an example.

There was longstanding animosity between the Judeans and Samaritans. It could be compared to that between the Palestinians and the Israelis today. This parable provocatively overthrows the negative stereotypes that the Jews held with regards to the Samaritans, and throws into question the conventional distinction between "us" and "them." A Samaritan who goes to the aid of a person, probably a Judean, who has been assaulted and left for dead, after two representatives of the established religion have ignored him, has stepped across a social and religious boundary. Jesus' Judean audience is forced to look through the eyes of the victim in the ditch, at their historic enemy, and to transcend social boundaries. Their neighbor includes other ethnic groups. A new social order is envisaged. God's Kingdom includes everyone.

Compare this to the Siddha Tirumular's famous saying:

"The whole of humanity is one family and the Lord we worship is Only One."

It is indeed ironic that Jesus' message of love your neighbor no matter who or what he is, and love God as your Self, was replaced by the message of the Christian Church: fear God, and condemn those who do not agree with your interpretation of Christianity. How much war, how much human suffering has occurred in the name of religion? The sayings of Jesus do not express religion's need to define truth or how to win salvation from God, nor to distinguish its believers from others. His spiritual teachings transcend all religions. They expand one's consciousness into a new egoless perspective.

Today, when the world is indeed a global village, thanks to the Internet, the media, the globalization of the economy and supersonic air travel, we are indeed many communities of interest. We can no longer ignore our neighbors.

When like the Good Samaritan, we take care of our neighbors; we may be surprised to find God as well. There is so much suffering in the world today. Is it not there so that we can learn to be compassionate, to go beyond "my" and "mine," and realize our true universal self? But in helping to relieve the suffering of others, it is important to meet them where they are, not where we want them to be. Too often, Christian missionaries seek to convert others to their way of thinking, in the guise of charitable service. This cultural imperialism ignores the values which other cultures cherish, and assumes that "we alone have the truth." The Good Samaritan did not try to convert the injured man. He had no ulterior motive, no agenda. The Lord has created everyone, and when we value the "unity in diversity" of his creation, we really pay homage to the Lord.

CHAPTER 6

What Did Jesus Not Say?

In chapter one, it was shown how modern historical research has determined that most of the teachings and statements attributed to Jesus in the four Gospels were not his own, but rather interpolations by anonymous authors. In chapter four we traced the development of early Christianity, which further obscured the original teachings of Jesus. There, we described how and why the proto-Orthodox Christians, beginning with Paul, replaced the teachings of Jesus with a highly organized church and religious dogma about Jesus as a personal Savior for all mankind. The good news that Jesus brought in his teachings, that the Kingdom of God is here, and how to enter it, with love and forgiveness, was replaced by the threat of eternal damnation if one did not accept Jesus Christ as ones personal savior.

In this chapter, we will discuss some of the aphorisms and sayings that come from level two or three analysis: those which are interpolations (words attributed to him, but probably originated with unknown evangelists) and those which definitely originated with others. While the list is not definitive, it may serve to illustrate the teachings of Christianity, as distinct from the teachings of Jesus. We will compare and contrast these teachings of Christianity with the teachings of the Yoga Siddhas. Some commentary as to the rules of evidence that helped to determine the status of these sayings will also be given.

Gospel of John

There was an overwhelming consensus among the scholars of the Jesus Seminar that the text of the Gospel of John, the Epistles of Paul, Acts and Revelation, contained few words that could be attributed to Jesus. Rather, they were most likely to be the words of the early church evangelists who taught that the person of Jesus was "the message," and that one needed to accept him as one's Savior in order to enter the Kingdom of Heaven on the Judgment Day.

Jesus never said that he was a savior, a messiah, or anything more than "the son of man." He never preached to others that they must see him as their Savior. This figure of Christ, which was developed by Paul in his new religion, was based upon the literary figure of Jesus created in the narratives about the life of Jesus in the Gospels. The words attributed to Jesus, particularly in the Gospel of John, portray Jesus as a mystic, and are highly spiritual. However, they are expressed in a context that attempts to convince the reader to adhere to the dogmas of the early churches, which were attempting to organize their beliefs and membership, and refute those of the Gnostics and others.

As we have seen in the chapter on "Modern Historical Research of Jesus and Early Christianity," "the two portraits of Jesus," that of the Synoptic Gospels and that of the Gospel of John, cannot both be historically accurate. The three "Synoptic Gospels" together with that of Thomas provide a "common view" of Jesus that is at great variance with that provided by John. Bear in mind, that none of the authors of the Gospels were apostles of Jesus. They were well educated, anonymous early Christians, writing in Greek between 35 and 70 years after the crucifixion of Jesus. The author of the Gospel of John, was probably a well educated Jew, who lived in Smyrna, in Asia Minor, now Turkey.

The Siddha yogis would point to the essential unity behind the contradictions in the "two portraits of Jesus." For the Siddhas, a mystic is however not someone who would ever call himself a savior, a messiah, for a mystic does not identify himself with his personality, his body nor his mission in life. Only a disciple might attempt to define their teacher in such a way.

A true mystic, which Jesus undoubtedly was, is one who experiences God impersonally, not as an object, but as Truth Consciousness, as *sat chit ananda,* (absolute existence, consciousness, bliss). This experience of *satchitananda* is an experience of the Lord in his Infinite state, the state of Love, the *summa bonnum*, what the Siddhas called *civam* (literally "goodness"), the supreme abstraction, which is behind all that exists, yet is above all relationships. This conception of a Supreme Being therefore transcends the world of relations, including any possible one with the man Jesus. However, It expresses Itself in an Ideal that has harmonized *satchitananda* within Itself. Jesus was such an Ideal. Jesus Christ is an archetypal Ideal of this Supreme Abstraction. The truth of *satchitananda* lies behind the imperfect reality of human existence. Jesus transcended his imperfect human state and harmonized his being, when the perfect supreme spirit revealed Itself to him. The ordinary mind of man can never reach such heights of realization of the Absolute.

The ordinary mind is incapable of such infinite realization because it is focused on only one object, sensory or abstract, at a time. But the Siddhas would say that a mystic like Jesus had transcended his ordinary mind to an expanded state of awareness free of all divisions, without the clash of ideas and egoism ("I am the body, I am angry, or hungry," etc.); the Infinite Mind is pure omnipresent, omnipotent Knowledge.

The Yoga Siddhas would affirm that it is this state of consciousness, attained by Jesus, which transcends the ordinary state, that is indeed the way to salvation, the way to the Kingdom of Heaven, to God-realization. It is not the man the world knows as Jesus, but the consciousness embodied in that man. It is through that Consciousness that we can be saved.

The "I am" Sayings

In John's Gospel, written after the others, about 90 C.E., Jesus frequently speaks of Himself in the first person, using the emphatic phrase I AM (Greek: *ego eimi*). This expression was widely used in the Greco-Roman world, and would have been recognized by the readers of the Gospel of John readers as an established formula in speech attributed to one of the gods. The author may even be alluding to the famous revelation of God in Exodus 3.14: "I am that I am."

There are no "I am" sayings in the other Gospels. Nor do they have any basis in the aphorisms, sage retorts and parables of the historical Jesus that appear in the other Gospels. They are the words of an evangelist addressing a community of early Christians, who shared his views, attempting to define itself in terms derived from the Scriptures, and to exclude those who do not share its viewpoints.

These sayings are significant in the *Samkhya* and yogic philosophies as "I am" expresses the realization of the Supreme Being at the limit of its objectivity and subjectivity. The sayings below reflect the teachings of the Siddhas. That of the fundamental Truth or reality of the Absolute, underlying the whole manifestation of the world, the Being, Conscious Bliss. And that, of the dynamic power behind creation, the "Becoming," the Supreme Energy. Through such sayings, we are guided toward an inner movement, toward the secret part of our selves, an inner being, a soul, inner mind, an inner life of budding growth and potential rebirth into a new Universal Life.

The best known "I am" sayings in John are:

"I am the bread of life" (6.35)

"I am the light of the world" (8.12)

"I existed before there was an Abraham" (8.58)

"I am the good shepherd" (10.11)

"I am resurrection and life" (11.25)

"I am the way, and I am truth, and I am life" (14.6)

"I am the authentic vine" (15.1)

From the beginning of this Gospel, readers are told who Jesus is and what he is. This is not the language typical of Jesus as found in the Synoptic Gospels, but it is typical of the language of the evangelist, someone who is trying to convert his listeners to the new Christian religion. The evangelist has replaced the teachings of Jesus with teachings about Jesus, as Lord and Savior. In the other Gospels, Jesus speaks of himself only rarely, and even then, with great humility. In this fourth Gospel, Jesus speaks constantly of himself and in elevated terms, and tells no parables. It is a language far removed from the one who spoke the parables and aphorisms.

The scholars of the Jesus Seminar saw a major theme dominating these sayings: access to the Father is through Jesus alone:

"If you love me, you'll obey my instructions. At my request the Father will provide you with yet another advocate, the authentic spirit, who will be with you forever." (John 14.15-17)

Love requires that one "accepts" and "obeys" Jesus' instructions, but where is Jesus' message of unconditional love, cutting across all social boundaries. In saying that no one may have access to God except through Him, the author of the Gospel of John contradicts the other Gospels, including Luke (see 11.52) and Thomas, wherein Jesus teaches his listeners how to enter into the Kingdom of heaven.

Can this statement of John be better understood in light of the teachings of the Yoga Siddhas? The "authentic spirit," "another advocate," is known in the Siddhas terminology as "the divine soul or the special Self." With reference to the detailed discussion about the role of the "Guru," at the end of the first chapter, according to the Yoga Siddhas, "Guru, God and Self are one." But how is one to distinguish the "inner guru," or guide or "authentic spirit?" One needs an external guide initially, and Jesus would be referring to this when he said "if you love me, you'll obey my instructions." That is, his teachings, his instructions are the external guru or guide. By following them one is turned inward and to hear the "inner guru," the "authentic spirit," and pure enough to distinguish its promptings from those of the ego.

The Farewell Prayer

Towards the end of the Gospels of John, Jesus is reported to have said: "Father, the time has come to honor your son, so your son may honor you. Just as you have given him authority over all humankind, so he can award real life to everyone you have given him. This real life: to know you as the one true God, and Jesus Christ, the one you sent...I have passed on your instructions to them, so the world hated them because they are aliens in the world... I also made your name known to them and will continue to make it known, so the kind of love you have for me may be theirs, and I may be theirs also." (John 17 1-25) (translation from *The Five Gospels: What Did Jesus Really Say?* pages 457-458)

This farewell speech had an enormous influence in the church's definition of the relation between Jesus and the Father in the fourth and fifth centuries C.E. and in many ways it provides a summary of the fourth Gospel's understanding of the message and mission of Jesus. It looks back on the success of the Church, its need for unity, as well as its alienation from the world. Nothing in it can be traced back to the aphorisms, parables or sage retorts of Jesus remembered in the other Gospels. It is characteristic of the phrases, theology and formulations characteristic of the fourth Gospel.

However, from the perspective of the teachings of the Yoga Siddhas, the issues raised in the speech, can be understood in a deeper sense. First, the name of "Jesus Christ" affirmed in this passage, is referring in a deeper sense, to the flow of God's power and grace. The "authority over all humankind" comes from the quality and character embodied in the human, known as Jesus, which arose out of his consciousness. It is the consciousness of Jesus, which enabled Jesus to know God, "(know you as the one true God)," which distinguishes him from the ordinary human. It is also what Jesus promised to make known to all who would believe: "so the kind of love you have for me may be theirs, and I may be theirs also."

Second, how to know God? God is infinite consciousness, but within that Infinite is the finite, envisaged and prefigured in form. The passage makes it clear that there is a co-existence of the Infinite and the finite, which is the very nature of the universal being. These co-exist analogously to the relationship between light and the Sun. The finite is the manifest aspect and the self-determining aspect of the Infinite, but the finite cannot exist in or by itself, it exists by the Infinite and is of one essence with the Infinite. God is time-less and space-less and is self-existent and is indefinable and can express Himself in all that ever exists at any point in time or space. God cannot be known in the ordinary sense of knowing a finite object. God is the ultimate subject, according to the Yoga Siddhas, the Eternal Witness of all creation. But one can become conscious of God, by becoming conscious of what is conscious within each of us. Through his parables, Jesus shows us how.

The End of the World

Jesus was a follower of John the Baptist, and was baptized by him in the river Jordan. But he eventually rejected the assertions of John the Baptist that the end of the world was at hand, as well as his asceticism. Jesus returned to urban areas to consort with common sinners, like tax collectors, outcasts, and the sick. Many of Jesus' early disciples had been disciples of John the Baptist, so after Jesus had gone, they returned to their former belief system, centered on the end of the world scenarios. This was elaborated in the early Christianity as eschatological doctrines, most notably in the Revelations of John, which predicted a Judgment Day, where all sinners would be cast into hell for eternity. This was certainly not the teaching of Jesus in the parables and aphorisms of the oral tradition, or even the Synoptic Gospels, nor of Thomas. It was not "the good news," which Jesus shared, that "the Kingdom of Heaven" is present all around us, and how to enter it while living, by purifying one's consciousness.

Here again, the issue regarding the "end of the world" can be better understood in light of the teachings of the Yoga Siddhas. The Siddhas teach that man's aim in each lifetime is evolution towards the realization of God, and those who do not evolve, devolve. The Siddhas teach that man must know himself and the world by going beyond his physical and mental surface nature, egoism, delusion and the consequences of his past thoughts, words and deeds, which is karma. He must come to know his true Self, his soul and the power and movement of the universe and the powers that control the world. He must come into communion with the divine spirit and become attuned to His Supreme Will and raise himself in purification and perfection into the Kingdom of Heaven, ever here on earth.

Similarly, the Siddhas would see that the Book of Revelations, the ultimate expression of the New Testament's vision of the end of the world, should not be taken literally, but as a metaphoric expression of the timeless five functions of the Lord: creation, preservation, destruction, obscuration and grace. These five functions are similarly and metaphorically represented in the iconic Nataraja, Dancing Shiva. The universe is due to His dynamic motion; energy moving outward into action, energy at work, conceptual, mechanical, spiritual, metnal, vital or material. It is only Shiva's lifted leg which keeps the world in motion. If His leg falls the universe dissolves, and returns to the static, immobile, silent, Eternal Reality.

Jesus' Dying Words

The Synoptic Gospels and John attribute a great variety of words from the Old Testament (Psalms 69.21, Job 19.25-27) to Jesus in his dying moments. As discussed in chapter four, these linked him to the old religion of Judaism, providing him legitimacy in the eyes of Gentiles, who valued what was old, and who did not trust what was new. The great variety in these attributions illustrates again how freely the individual evangelists put words of scripture on the lips of Jesus.[1] False attribution or interpolation, as it is referred to by scholars, served the purposes of the evangelists, who sought to "Christianize" Jesus and to link him to Old Testament prophecies, claiming that he was fulfilling these.

At the Tomb

The words ascribed to Jesus in his encounter with Mary at the empty tomb, John 20.15-17 are credited to the storyteller. The various accounts of what was said, by different evangelists, reveals the storytellers art. None of the sayings are memorable or expressed the manner in which Jesus spoke.

Doubting Thomas

As discussed in chapter four's section entitled "The Gospel of John versus the Gospels of Thomas, Matthew, Mark and Luke," John is the only Gospel to report the incident wherein Jesus appeared to the disciples after his crucifixion, and admonished Thomas for "doubting" that he had risen until Thomas had touched his wounds. It is typical of the Gospel of John to reprimand and even ridicule those who must literally see to believe; only those who believe without having to "see" are blessed, according to John.

The Gospel of John affirmed that only by faith in Jesus Christ as one personal savior could one be saved. No other Gospel says anything like this. As we have discussed earlier, the author of the Gospel of John sought to discredit Thomas because of the Gnostic teachings in the Gospel of Thomas affirmed what John denied: that one could have a direct and intimate relationship with God through inner knowing.[2]

The Familiar Tenets of Christianity Cannot Be Traced to Jesus Himself

Among the most important things which Christianity claims, but which in fact Jesus never said are the following:

- Jesus made no claim to be the anointed Messiah, or one's Savior, or to be an incarnation of God. He always referred to himself as the "son of man," out of great modesty. There is a near universal consensus among scholars that at the time of Jesus, this expression was in general usage in Galilean Aramaic both as a noun (meaning "a human being") and as a substitute for the indefinite pronoun and as a periphrasis for "I."[3]

- Jesus made no predictions of an apocalyptic end of the world, nor about a coming judgment. He made no prediction of his second coming.

- Jesus made no claims that he was dying for the sins of others nor that sins are forgiven by believing in him. He did not forgive the sins of others or authorize anyone to do so. He made no claim that salvation comes to those who believed that his death on the cross is their redemption. Such claims came from Paul, and later from the anonymous author of the Gospel of John.

- Jesus announced no fulfillment of Old Testament prophecy.

- Jesus made no claim to be the only "Son of God." "Son of God" was a designation created by evangelists who sought to link him to King David, as this is a term reserved for kings, who derive their authority from God, and who sought to exalt him as the figure of Christ, with a unique relationship to God.[4] The capitalization of the "s" in "Son" was made when the Bible was translated from Greek into English in the 17th Century. There are no capital letters in Greek.

- Jesus founded no church; he did not appoint Peter or any other disciple to do so. He made no claims of infallibility for himself or others. He never attempted to force anyone to follow him, nor threatened anyone with damnation if they did not.

- Jesus never promised the coming and constancy of the "Holy Spirit." He never claimed that this "Holy Spirit" would tell the authors of the Bible what to write.

- Jesus never wrote a Gospel, nor did he ask anyone else to do so.

- Jesus never claimed to have been the product of a virgin birth.

- Jesus never asked anyone not to observe the Jewish Laws. He frequently interpreted the law and admonished his listeners to realize and follow its deeper sense.
- Not a single word written by Paul in the Epistles, (most of the New Testament, revered by Christians) gives the actual teachings of Jesus, nor do they mention even one of his parables. The teachings of Jesus were completely distinct from those of Paul, whose Epistles were his own ideas.
- Jesus did not teach fear of death and fear of damnation for sins. His were joyous tidings. Paul, however, transformed "the good news" into threatening news, and taught repeatedly that all are subject to the wrath of God, (Ephesians 2.3) quite lost (Romans 5.18, Corinthians 15.18) without hope and without God, (Ephesians 2.12) for Satan has power over everyone (without exception). (Romans 3.9, Galatians 3.22, Colossians 2.14) A sentence of damnation hangs like a sword of Damocles over all people. (Romans 5.16) Paul established a religion of fear and threats.
- Jesus did not teach, as Paul did, that the human individual can do nothing himself to secure salvation, (Romans 3.24, 3.28, 9.11, 9.16, 1 Corinthians 1.29) (Galatians 2.16) nor that only Grace can save one. Jesus did not teach, as Paul did, that only by joining the fold, and converting to Christianity, would salvation would come automatically.
- Jesus did not teach that, however exemplary and good his or her life may have been, one is damned for eternity, if he or she does not gratefully acknowledge his sacrifice on the cross as constituting their entire personal salvation. This central teaching of Christianity finds no place in the Gospels, or in the Sermon on the Mount or in any of the parables or aphorisms of Jesus, or even in the Lord's Prayer. If Jesus believed that his sacrificial death was so important to the salvation of mankind, he would have said so. But he never did.

Not only did Jesus not say the above. Neither did his direct disciples. As we have seen, none of the twenty seven books in the New Testament Canon were written by a direct disciple of Jesus. Furthermore, many sayings of Jesus, in the Gospel of Thomas, considered by scholars to be authentic, were kept out of the New Testament. Was it because it did not conform to the Orthodox views that only by believing in Jesus Christ as Lord and savior one can find salvation? Its recent discovery has provided impetus to the moral imperative to reform Christian dogma.

Christianity Was Founded by Paul

The Church historian Wilhelm Nestle went so far as to say: "Christianity is the religion founded by Paul; it replaced Christ's gospel with a gospel about Christ."[5] Holger Kersten has charged that "Paulinism in this sense means a misinterpretation and indeed counterfeiting of Christ's actual teachings, as arranged and initiated by Paul... by building on the belief of salvation through the expiatory death of God's first-born, Paul regressed to the primitive Semitic religions of earlier times, in which parents were commanded to give up their first-born in a bloody sacrifice. Paul also prepared the path for the later ecclesiastical teachings on original sin and the trinity... Paul disregarded many teachings of Jesus; instead, he placed Jesus upon a pedestal and turned him into the Christ figure that Jesus never intended to be. If it is ever possible to discover any profound knowledge or truth in the heart of Christianity, it will only be by rejecting obvious counterfeits that have been considered so sacrosanct as to be untouchable, and by turning to the true pure teachings of Jesus and the real essence of Religion."[6]

Paul was largely responsible for basing early Christian theology on the belief in Jesus Christ as the sole means of personal salvation. It is indeed ironic and contradictory that Paul, a great mystic, developed a theology that ignored the spiritual, even mystical teachings of Jesus' parables, and condemned other paths including "inner knowing," and affirmed that by faith in Jesus Christ alone one is saved. It is even more ironic, as we have seen, that he reserved higher mystical teachings for his most worthy students. In seeking to bring the teachings of Jesus to those who were not

Jews, he freed Christians from following the Jewish law, by emphasizing the special personage of Jesus. In so doing he replaced the teachings of Jesus with a religion about Jesus. He struck a sympathetic chord, however, for it is far easier to worship someone "perfect" than to follow their admonition: "Be ye perfect."

Consequences of Christianity Replacing the Teachings of Jesus

The tenets of Christianity, summarized above, replaced the original teachings of Jesus, as described in the previous chapter. The consequences for Western civilization and the so called "third world" ever since, have been immense. By creating an artificial division between themselves and others, Christians have fomented numerous religious wars, including the Crusades, the medieval conflicts between Protestants and Catholics, anti-Semitism culminating in the Holocaust, and have even justified in the name of religion the extermination of whole cultures during colonial campaigns in Africa, the Americas, and Asia. Christianity became a proselytizing religion, whose members claim that it is their duty, indeed their right to convert others to their way of thinking, using violence, even murder if necessary. Conversion campaigns by Christian missionaries are rampant today in India, Africa, Americas and Asia, even though they violate the universally recognized human rights of religious freedom of those who are their targets. The subjugation and disenfranchisement of women in Western society was justified in the name of Christian religion. At one time, even slavery was justified by it.

Untold millions of Christians down through the centuries have been indoctrinated with the belief that "I am a sinner, and there is nothing which I can do to escape eternal suffering in hell unless I accept Jesus as my personal savior." Fear of God has replaced love for God in their psyche. Guilt, suppression of desires, internal division, skepticism and the glorification of suffering as imaged by Jesus on the cross has replaced the message of forgiveness, compassion, simplicity, truth, love, self-discipline, self-purification, detachment from materialistic desires, the presence of the Kingdom of God, mystical communion with it, and perfection which Jesus brought as his "good news."

While human nature could possibly have found another belief system to justify its egoistic, fearful tendencies if Christianity had not survived, we can only imagine how Western civilization might have evolved had the original teachings of Jesus been promulgated by Christian communities.

Conclusions and Recommendations

1. The discoveries of ancient manuscripts, and their analysis by independent critical scholars using scientific methods provide much insight into the original wisdom teachings of Jesus.
2. Study of the of the often enigmatic parables and sayings of Jesus in light of the Yoga Siddhas is revealing and enlightening.
3. The "sayings" and parables of Jesus are remarkably similar to those of the Yoga Siddhas. The wisdom teachings of both Jesus and the Yoga Siddhas are essentially the same. They both point to states of realization which, everyone, according to Jesus and the Siddhas, can and should aspire to. Jesus referred to this state of realization as the "Kingdom of God." The Siddhas referred to it as samadhi (cognitive absorption) and prescribed the methods of Kundalini Yoga. The wisdom teachings of Jesus and the Yoga Siddhas both referred to the obstacles to its realization, as ignorance, delusion, and egoism. They taught that to attain it, one must apply methods of spiritual discipline and self-purification, to transcend the ordinary egoistic perspective.
4. The Apostles Matthew, Mark, Luke and John were not the authors of the four canonical Gospels, and so their narratives of what Jesus did are not eyewitness accounts, which can be relied upon with any degree of assurance. They were written by anonymous evangelists of disparate early Christian churches, three to five decades after the crucifixion of Jesus.

5. The "sayings" and parables of Jesus, circulated orally during the first decades following his crucifixion before being recorded, are probably the most authentic source of his teachings that we have available today. What Jesus really said (in the canonical Gospels and in the "sayings" of the Gospel of Thomas), is probably limited to a few dozen parables, aphorisms and sharp retorts. To these "sayings" many other things were attributed to Jesus by those who were attempting to define who Jesus was and to interpret His teachings.
6. In the Gospels of Matthew, Mark and Luke:
a. Jesus emphasized that the Kingdom of God was accessible to us here and now. He taught that by overcoming one's ignorance of it, and by self-discipline and purification of desires and attachments, one could experience it in this life in the world.
b. Jesus taught that God has unconditional love for all of humanity, not only those who believe that Jesus is God's "only begotten son" and personal savior.
c. Jesus never taught that "no one could come to the Father except by me." Rather, He challenged his listeners to transform their condition into a means of purification. He taught that one could enter God's Kingdom through reflecting deeply and gaining insight on the inner meaning in his parables, doing the opposite of what human nature demands, becoming pure and loving.
7. The wisdom teachings of Jesus were replaced with a religion about Jesus, by early Christian evangelists, beginning with Paul and the author of the Gospel of John, and subsequently by those who, over the next three centuries defined Church dogma and Church authority, and who declared other forms of Christianity as heretical.
8. Christianity was not created by Jesus, nor was He responsible for any division between Judaism and Christianity, nor for any sectarianism.
9. Modern biblical scholarship reveals that there are "two portraits" of Jesus in the four canonical gospels: that of a wisdom teacher of parables, who rarely speaks of himself, and never in elevated terms, never claiming to be a savior, nor to forgive the sins of others, as described in the synoptic (parallel) Gospels of Matthew, Mark and Luke, and

secondly, Jesus Christ, as described in the Gospel of John, who promises salvation to those who believe that "he" is the Savior of all mankind, and condemns all others to eternal damnation.

We can reconcile these two portraits of Jesus by interpreting them in light of what is referred to the Yoga Siddha literature as "the inner Guru." The Yoga Siddhas say that there is an inner Guru, a secret soul in all of us. A veiled presence, burns in the temple of our heart of hearts, behind the conditioning of our ignorant mind, body and life. This flame of the Godhead (Jesus) is kept lit even if we do not consciously keep it burning through knowledge, love or worship. This flame is born with us and out of God. It is the hidden guide and inspiration. It is both our wisdom guide and our "Savior."

Recommendations

This book records my own personal search for the historical Jesus and his authentic teachings, and is far from being a manifesto. It has had no forgone objectives or hypotheses to prove, other than to identify the original, authentic teachings of Jesus and to compare them with those of the Yoga Siddhas. Having arrived at the above conclusions, however, I feel moved to make the following recommendations:

1. That people of faith not ignore reason, and support the research and dissemination of the findings of scholars who continue to reveal the paths to truth created by the saints, sages and Siddhas of all times.
2. That scholars of comparative religion, early Christianity and Yoga, conduct much more research into the mystical practices common to early Christianity and classical Yoga and tantra.
3. That practical spiritual disciplines, new ethics and new language which is inspired by the original wisdom teachings of Jesus be considered and adopted in place of those which are not based upon his authentic teachings.
4. That everyone seek inspiration in the wisdom teachings of saints, sages and Siddhas, recognizing that human survival and civilization is

threatened by many crises, in part due to divisions created by religion, language, property, competition, and globalization.
5. May Christians of all denominations replace their commitment to sectarian and doctrinal divisions with a commitment to the spiritual discipline of Jesus.
6. May Christians become disciples of Jesus and His wisdom teachings.
7. May a religion of "love thy neighbor" become universal.
8. May everyone aspire for the realization of "the Kingdom of Heaven" within and here in this world through surrender of the ego consciousness and transformation of human nature.
9. May everyone realize Divine perfection through a progressive process of purification inspired by the wisdom teachings and disciplines of Jesus and the Yoga Siddhas.

NOTES

Introduction

1. *Faith and Reason*, page 1, paragraphs 1-2

Chapter 1: Modern Historical Research of Jesus and Early Christianity

1. Letter to John Adams, January 24, 1814, cited in *The Gospel According to Jesus*, pages 4-5
2. *The Gospel According to Jesus*, page 4
3. *The Five Gospels: What Did Jesus Really Say?*, page 5
4. *The Five Gospels, What Did Jesus Really Say*, page 5
5. *The Five Gospels: What Did Jesus Really Say?*, pages 5-6
6. *The Five Gospels: What did Jesus Really Say?*, page 6
7. *The Five Gospels: What Did Jesus Really Say?*, page 10
8. *The Five Gospels: What Did Jesus Really Say?*, page 11
9. *The Five Gospels: What Did Jesus Really Say?*, pages 10-11
10. *The Five Gospels: What Did Jesus Really Say?*, pages 16-25
11. *Beyond Belief*, page 45
12. *The Five Gospels: What Did Jesus Really Say?*, page 25
13. *The Five Gospels: What Did Jesus Really Say?*, page 26
14. *The Five Gospels: What Did Jesus Really Say?*, page 28
15. *The Five Gospels: What Did Jesus Really Say?*, page 28
16. *The Five Gospels: What Did Jesus Really Say?*, page 29
17. *The Five Gospels: What Did Jesus Really Say?*, pages 31-32
18. *The Five Gospels: What Did Jesus Really Say?*, page 32

Notes

Chapter 2: Paradoxical Teachings of the God-men

1. *The Guru Function*, page 5
2. *The Yoga of Jesus: Reflections about its Historical Roots,* page 5
3. *The Yoga of Tirumular: Essays on the Tirumandiram*, page 232
4. *The Yoga of the Eighteen Siddhas: An Anthology*, pages 11-45
5. *Yoga, Immortality and Freedom*, page 302
6. *The Yoga of Siddha Boganathar*, Volume 1, pages 2-4
7. *The Yoga of Siddha Boganathar,* Volume 1, page 5
8. *The Yoga of Siddha Boganathar,* Volume 1, page 10
9. *The Yoga of Siddha Boganathar*, Volume 1, page 11
10. *The Yoga of the Eighteen Siddhas: An Anthology*, pages 242-243
11. *The Yoga of the Eighteen Siddhas: An Anthology*, page 143
12. *The Yoga of Siddha Boganathar,* Volume 1, page 12
13. *The Oxford Companion to the Bible*, page 61
14. *Babaji and the 18 Siddha Kriya Yoga Tradition*, page 90
15. *The Yoga of Siddha Boganathar*, Volume 1, page 19
16. *The Yoga of Siddha Boganathar*, Volume 1, pages 18-19
17. *Kriya Yoga Sutras of Patanjali and the Siddhas*, I.24, page 31
18. *The Historical Jesus*, pages 311-312
19. *Autobiography of a Yogi*
20. *The Yoga of Siddha Boganathar*, Volume 1, page 13
21. *The Yoga of Siddha Boganathar*, Volume 1, page 14
22. *The Yoga of Siddha Boganathar*, Volume 1, page 27
23. *Kriya Yoga Sutras of Patanjali and the Siddhas*, pages 94-95
24. *Gospel of Judas*, pages 21-23
25. *Gospel of Judas*, pages 33-34

Chapter 3: The Gospel of Thomas: A Gnostic Text?

1. *The Other Bible*, page 299
2. *The Other Bible*, pages 464-481
3. *The Five Gospels: What Did Jesus Really Say?,* page 474
4. *The Gospel of Thomas*, page 10
5. *The Gnostic Gospels*, page xxxiii

6. *The Gospel of Thomas*, page 112
7. *Kriya Yoga Sutras of Patanjali and the Siddhas*, pages 2-3
8. *Kriya Yoga Sutras of Patanjali and the Siddhas*, pages 185-186
9. *The Glossary of Terms*, page 228
10. *Kriya Yoga Sutras of Patanjali and the Siddhas*, pages 2-4, 13
11. *The Gnostic Gospels*, page 148
12. *The Historical Jesus*, pages 421-422
13. *The Gospel of Thomas*, page 113
14. *Kriya Yoga Sutras of Patanjali and the Siddhas*, pages 221-222
15. *Kriya Yoga Sutras of Patanjali and the Siddhas*, page 128
16. *Kriya Yoga Sutras of Patanjali and the Siddhas*, page 57
17. *The Gospel of Thomas*, page 116
18. *The Gnostic Gospels*, page 148
19. *The Gnostic Gospels*, pages 138-140
20. *The Gnostic Gospels*, page 15
21. *The Gnostic Gospels*, pages 135-140

Chapter 4: Early Christianity: the Formation of the Church and its Dogma

1. *The Jesus Papers*, pages 251-261
2. *Oxford Companion to the Bible*, pages 6-10
3. *Lost Christianities*, pages 171-172
4. *Lost Christianities*, page 92
5. *Lost Christianities*, page 92
6. *Lost Christianities*, page 15
7. *Lost Christianities*, page 15
8. *Lost Christianities*, pages 99-102
9. *Lost Christianities*, pages 106-109
10. *The Oxford Companion to the Bible*, page 256
11. *Lost Christianities*, page 115
12. *The Gnostic Gospels*, page 36
13. *Lost Christianities*, page 185
14. *Lost Christianities*, page 143
15. *Lost Christianities/Lost Scriptures*, page 193

16. *Lost Christianities*, pages 111-112
17. *Lost Christianities*, page 192
18. *On First Principles* 1:3, *Lost Christianities*, pages 153-155
19. *Lost Christianities*, page 180
20. *The Gnostic Gospels*, page 143
21. *Gnosticism*, page 942
22. *Gospel of Thomas*, pages 27-30
23. *The Gnostic Gospels*, page 145
24. *The Gnostic Gospels*, pages 164-165
25. *Kriya Yoga Sutras of Patanjali and the Siddhas*, page 20
26. *The Gnostic Gospels*, page 146
27. *The Study of the History of Religion,* Volume 1, page 349
28. *The Gnostic Gospels*, page 149
29. *Lost Christianities*, page 194
30. *Beyond Belief: the Secret Gospel of Thomas*, page 34
31. *Beyond Belief: the Secret Gospel of Thomas*, pages 36-37
32. *Beyond Belief: the Secret Gospel of Thomas*, page 58
33. *Beyond Belief: the Secret Gospel of Thomas*, pages 66-67
34. *Beyond Belief: the Secret Gospel of Thomas*, pages 70-71
35. *Lost Christianities*, pages 230-231
36. *Lost Christianities*, pages 234-235
37. *Lost Christianities*, page 231
38. *Lost Christianities*, page 245
39. *Lost Christianities*, pages 242-244
40. *Lost Christianities*, pages 248-251

Chapter 5: What Did Jesus Really Say?

1. *The Five Gospels: What Did Jesus Really Say?*, page 144
2. *Babaji and the 18 Siddha Kriya Yoga Tradition*, page 141
3. *The Five Gospels: What Did Jesus Really Say?*, pages 484-485
4. *The Five Gospels: What Did Jesus Really Say?*, page 195
5. *The Five Gospels: What Did Jesus Really Say?*, page 531
6. *The Five Gospels: What Did Jesus Really Say?*, page 223
7. *The Five Gospels: What Did Jesus Really Say?*, page 223

8. *The Five Gospels: What Did Jesus Really Say?*, page 138
9. *Kriya Yoga Sutras of Patanjali and the Siddhas*, page 109
10. *Kriya Yoga Sutras of Patanjali and the Siddhas*, page xxvi
11. *Kriya Yoga Sutras of Patanjali and the Siddhas*, page 70
12. *The Five Gospels: What Did Jesus Really Say?*, page 69
13. *Kriya Yoga Sutras of Patanjali and the Siddhas*, page 99
14. *The Five Gospels: What Did Jesus Really Say?*, pages 152-153
15. *Kriya Yoga Sutras of Patanjali and the Siddhas*, pages 2-4
16. *The Five Gospels: What Did Jesus Really Say?*, page 155
17. *The Practice of Integral Yoga*, page 42
18. *The Five Gospels*, pages 56-57
19. *The Yoga of Siddhar Boganathar*, Volume 1, page 208
20. *The Five Gospels: What Did Jesus Really Say?*, page 307
21. *The Yoga of Siddha Boganathar*, Volume 1, pages 11-12
22. *The Five Gospels: What Did Jesus Really Say?*, page 325
23. *The Five Gospels: What Did Jesus Really Say?*, page 149
24. *The Five Gospels: What Did Jesus Really Say?*, pages 356-357
25. *The Gospel of Jesus*, pages 36-38
26. *The Yoga of Siddha Tirumular*, page 62
27. *The Yoga of Siddha Tirumular*, pages 62-63
28. *The Five Gospels: What Did Jesus Really Say?*, page 358-359
29. *The Five Gospels: What Did Jesus Really Say?*, page 196

Chapter 6: What Did Jesus Not Say?

1. *The Five Gospels: What Did Jesus Really Say?*, page 465
2. *The Five Gospels: What Did Jesus Really Say?*, page 467
3. *The Oxford Companion to the Bible*, page 712
4. *The Oxford Companion to the Bible*, pages 710-711
5. *Jesus Lived in India*, page 28
6. *Jesus Lived in India*, page 29

BIBLIOGRAPHY

Ahlund, Jan S., *The Grace of Babaji's Kriya Yoga: A course of lessons,* Babaji's Kriya Yoga and Publications, 2006

Barnstone, Willis, Editor, *The Other Bible: Jewish Pseudepigrapha, Christian Apocrypha, Gnostic Scriptures, Kabbalah, Dead Sea Scrolls*, HarperCollins, 1984.

Baigent, Michael, *The Jesus Papers,* HarperElement, 2006

Briggs, George Weston, *Goraknath and the Kanphata Yogis,* Motilal Banarsidass, 1938

Crossan, John Dominic, *The Historical Jesus: the Life of a Mediterranean Jewish Peasant,* HarperCollins, 1992.

Ehrman, Bart D. *Lost Christianities: The Battles for Scriputre and the Faiths We Never Knew,* Oxford University Press, 2003

Eliade, Mircea, *Yoga, Immortality and Freedom,* Princeton University Press, 1958

Feuerstein, Georg, *The Yoga Tradition: Its History, Literature, Philosophy and Practice,* Hohm Press, 1998

Feuerstein, Georg, *Holy Madness: The Shock Tactics and Radical Teachings of Crazy-Wise Adepts, Holy Fools, and Rascal Gurus,* Paragon House, 1991

Feuerstein, Georg, *Is Yoga a Religion,* unpublished paper, Yoga Research and Education Center, 2002, www.traditionalyogastudies.com

Feuerstein, Georg, *The Guru Function: Broadcasting Reality,* unpublished paper, Yoga Research and Education Center, 2002, www.traditionalyogastudies.com

Feuerstein, Georg, *The Yoga of Jesus: Reflections about its Historical Roots,* unpublished paper, Yoga Research and Education Center, 2003, www.traditionalyogastudies.com

Feuerstein, Georg, *The Deeper Dimension of Yoga,* Shamballa, 2003

Funk, Robert and Hoover, Roy W., *The Five Gospels: The Search for the Authentic Words of Jesus,* Harper Collins, 1993

Ganapathy, T.N., *The Yoga of Siddha Boganathar volume 1,* Babaji's Kriya Yoga and Publications, 2003.

Ganapathy, T.N., editor, *The Yoga of the Eighteen Siddha: An Anthology,* Babaji's Kriya Yoga and Publications, 2005

Ganapathy, T.N., *The Yoga of Siddha Tirumular: Essays on the Tirumandiram,* Babaji's Kriya Yoga and Publications, 2006

Govindan, Marshall, *Babaji and the 18 Siddha Kriya Yoga Tradition,* Babaji's Kriya Yoga and Publications, Inc. 1991

Govindan, Marshall, *Kriya Yoga Sutras of Patanjali and the Siddhas,* Babaji's Kriya Yoga and Publications, 2000

Govindan, Marshall, Editor, *Thirumandiram: A Classic of Yoga and Tantra,* by Siddha Thirumoolar, Babaji's Kriya Yoga and Publications, 1992

Kandaswamy, S.N., *The Yoga of Siddha Avvai,* Babaji's Kriya Yoga and Publications, 2005

Kasser, Rodolphe, Meyer, Marvin and Wurst, Gregor, *The Gospel of Judas,* National Geographic, 2006

Kersten, Holger, *Jesus lived in India: his unknown life before and after the crucifixion,* Element Books, Ltd.

Mack, Burton, *The Lost Gospel: The Book of Q and Christian Origins,* San Francisco, 1994.

Metzger, Bruce, and Coogan, Michael D. Editors, *The Oxford Companion to the Bible,* Oxford University Press, 1993

Meyer, Marvin and Bloom, Harold, *The Gospel of Thomas: The Hidden Sayings of Jesus,* Harper Collins 1992

Mitchell, Stephen, *The Gospel According to Jesus,* Harper Collins 1993

Muktibodhananda, Swami, *Hatha Yoga Pradipika,* Yoga Publications Trust, Bihar School of Yoga, 1985

Nock, A.D., The Study of the History of Religion, volume 1,

Pagels, Elaine, *Beyond Belief: the Secret Gospel of Thomas,* Vintage Books, Random House, 2000

Pagels, Elaine, *The Gnostic Gospels,* Vintage Books, Random House, 1979

Spong, John Shelby, *The Sins of Scripture: Exposing the Bible's Texts of Hate to Reveal the God of Love,* Harper Collins, 2005

T.S. Anantha Murthy, *Maharaj: A Biography of Shriman Tapasviji Maharaj, a Mahatma who lived for 185 Years*, The Dawn Horse Press, 1986

Satprem, *Sri Aurobindo, The Adventure of Consciousness, Institute for Evolutionary Research,* 1993

Sri Aurobindo, *Glossary of Terms*, Sri Aurobindo Ashram Press, 1975.

Vanmikanathan, G., *Pathway to God Trod by Saint Ramalingar*, Bhartiya Vidya Bhavan,1976.

Swami Prabhavananda's *The Sermon on the Mount According to Vedanta*, Vedanta Society, 1966.

Vatican website: www.vatican.va, *Papal Encyclical Faith and Reason.*

White, David Gordon, *The Alchemical Body: Siddh Traditions in Meieval India,* University of Chicago Press, 1996

Yogananda, Paramhansa Yogananda, *Autobiography of a Yogi*, The Philosophical Library, 1946. Reprint 1994 by Crystal Clarity, Publishers

Yogananda, Paramahansa, *The Second Coming of Christ*

Zvelebil, Kamil V., *The Poets of the Powers,* Integral Publishing, 1993. Distributed by Babaji's Kriya Yoga and Publications.

Glossary

Greek, Christian and Biblical Terms

1. Abba- Father
2. Aeons- everlasting, indefinite period of time
3. Allogenes- another race, or a stranger
4. Avesta- the sacred text of the early Persians
5. canonical - officially approved; orthodox; appearing in the Bible
6. chreia - from the Greek *chreiodes*, "useful"
7. Christian - from the Greek word *christos*, meaning "anointed one," with an ending meaning follower of, or partisan of. First used probably in Antioch by non-Jewish opponents, as a derogatory term, and to distinguish them from the Jews.
8. Confucius - Chinese sage and author of wise sayings, 500 B.C.E.
9. Codex Sinaiticus-volumes of scripture
10. Coptic-liturgical language of the Egyptian Christian Church
11. Council of Nicaea in 325 C.E- council, which created the formal statement of doctrine of the Christian faith.
12. Docetism - from the Greek word *doceo* – "appear" or "seem." Considered to be a heretical sect in the early Christian church believing Christ had no human form and only appeared to have died on the Cross.

13. Ebionites - early vegetarian Jewish Christians, who believed that Jesus was a perfect sacrifice to atone for humanity's sins; they followed all other Jewish practices, descended from the apostles Peter and James of the Jerusalem church.
14. Edict of Toleration - a proclamation by Roman Emperor Constantine in 313 C.E. ending the persecution of the Christians.
15. Ekklesias - assemblies, reference to early Christians
16. ennoia - internal reflection
17. Epinoia - Eucharist
18. Eschatological - the teaching concerning last things, such as the resurrection of the dead, the Last Judgment, the end of this world, and the creation of a new one, developed by the Old Testament prophets during the tenth to sixth centuries BCE, and later by early Christians waiting for the second coming of Christ.
19. Eschaton - last event, cataclysm, apocalypse
20. Essenes - an ascetic Jewish sect existing in ancient Palestine from the 2nd century B.C. to the 3rd century A.D. In 1948, at Qumram, near the Dead Sea, ancient manuscripts related to this sect were discovered.
21. Gnostic - possessing intellectual or spiritual knowledge, those who valued inquiry into spiritual truth above faith
22. Judean - the name for a native born person of what is now the southern part of modern day Israel, formerly Judea.
23. Marcionites - followers of the second century evangelist and theologian, Marcion, who rejected everything Jewish.
24. Messiah - derived from the Hebrew word *masiah*, meaning "anointed," most often used in the Hebrew bible in reference to the anointing of kings with oil. In Greek it is translated as *christos*, It denotes an expected or longed for savior, especially in the Jewish tradition.
25. Nag Hammadi - the place where over forty previously unknown documents related to early Christianity, together with several previ-

ously known ones, were discovered in 1945 in Upper Egypt, in a jar, buried in a cave. Many were Gnostic.

26. Pleroma – "Fullness," God's divine realm, referred to in the Gnostics myths as the origin of the world.
27. pronoia - anticipatory awareness, in Gnosticsm
28. proto-Orthodox - the theologians, church leaders and their followers to whom we owe the most familiar features of what is considered as Christianity today: four Gospels only, twenty-seven books in the New Testament, and included in this Canon of Orthodox Scripture, the Old Jewish Bible, as well as the church hierarchy, a set of doctrinal beliefs (Christ as both fully God and fully man; the sacred Trinity: Father, Son and Holy Spirit) and the sacraments of baptism and the Eucharist, marriage and death. Among the most important proto-orthodox theologians were Ignatius, Bishop of Antioch, at the beginning of the second century C.E., Polycarp, Irenaeus, Bishop of Lyon, Tertullian, and Origen.
29. Samaritan - the name for a native born person of the northern region of present day Israel, or Samaria.
30. Septuagint - the Greek Old Testament, a popular reference for early Christian theologians and Church leaders.
31. Stromata - an early Christian work refuting Gnosticism, written by Clement of Alexandria
32. Synoptic – "seen together," referring to the Gospels of Mark, Matthew and Luke, because of their close similarities, which permits the texts to be set out in parallel for comparison.
33. Zostrianos - the longest of the Gnostic texts, found at Nag Hammadi, which tells how one spiritual master attained enlightenment, implicitly setting out a program for others to follow, including meditation and purification of desires, reaching enlightenment.

Yoga Terms

A

ABHISEKA. Sprinkling of water as in a baptism or ritual bathing of a statue of a Deity.

ACHARYA. Preceptor a teacher or preceptor.

ADVAITIC. Non-duality, the Oneness of All.

AGNEYI YOGA DHARMA. The awakening of Kundalini Shakti.

AHIMSA. Non-harming in thought, word or deed.

ANBU. Pure love.

APARIGRAHAH. Greediness.

ARRUPADAI. Showing the path to others.

ASHRAM. A place of peace; the hermitage of yogis.

ASHTANGA YOGA. The path of eight limbs to realization.

ASMITA. I am-ness.

ASTEYA. Non-stealing.

ATMAN. The Transcendental Self.

AUMKARA. Chanting of the Divine sound, the primordial sound of the Universe.

AVIDYA. Ignorance of the truth.

B

BRAHMAN. The Supreme principle behind all things; universal divine power.

BRAHMACHARYA. A stage of life; the ideal of chastity as brahmic conduct.

BRAHMIN. Member of a Hindu society held in charge of the sacred knowledge.

C

CHAKRA. Subtle energy centers along the spinal cord, which affect physiological and psychic functions; a conjunction of nadis or subtle energy currents.

CINMAYA. Body of light.

CIT. Awareness or consciousness.

D

DARSHAN. Visions or witnessing.

DEVABHAJU. Followers of the *Vedic* faith or the worshippers of the *devas* or gods.

DIKSA. Initiation or moment of awakening of a mantra or of ones spiritual being.

DIVYA DEHA. Divine body, lustrous body.

DIYATE. Endowing knowledge.

DVIJA. Born-again, born anew in a spiritual body.

G

GURU. An authority of the greatest knowledge.

GURU PARAMPARA. The successive passing of spiritual knowledge from one guru to another within a spiritual lineage.

I

ISHVARA. Highest Lord; Supreme God or Personal God.

J

JIVA. "To live" the individual soul.

JIVAN MUKTI. Liberated soul while living in a human body.

JIYANTA MORA. Being "dead" in the world; liberated as a jivanmukti.

JNANA YOGA. A path toward the spiritual unfoldment of wisdom within an individual, the union with Knowledge.

K

KAIVALYAM. Absolute freedom and oneness, aloneness.

KAILAYA DEHA. Body of light; kailaya refers to the metaphorical abode of Siva on Mt Kailash.

KARMA. The impersonal principle of cause and effect, which shapes ones life; consequence.

KAYA SIDDHI. Process by which the body is transformed from a physical to a spiritual substance to attain immortality.

KOAN. A zen Buddhist riddle, or subject of contemplation.

KRIYA YOGA. Yoga of action; of constant practice, self-study and devotion to the Lord.

KSIYATE. Eliminating lower impulses.

KUNDALINI. Serpent Power; potential power and consciousness.

KUNDALINI YOGA. Yoga of awakening this potential power and raising it along the sushumna nadi to unite it with the Lord.

M

MANIPURA. "City of jewels;" solar plexus center of will-power.

MAYA. That, which emanates from Pure Consciousness, creating the appearance of a manifest universe.

MOKSHA. Liberation from the rounds of birth, death and rebirth.

MUKTI. Released from, liberated from the rounds of birth, death and rebirth.

N

NADIS. A subtle channel of energy within.

NANDI. "The joyful;" the mount of Lord Siva, the soul of man.

NIYAMAS. Restraints of behavior.

O

OLI UDAMBU. Body of light.

P

PATI. The Lord.
PASA. The fetters, obstacles.
PASU. The soul.
PRAJNA. Insight.
PRAKRITI. Nature.
PURUSHA. Supreme Consciousness.

R

RISHI. A yogic seer.

S

SAIVA SIDDHANTA. The final conclusions of Saivism; the divine revelations of the twenty-eight Saiva Agamas.

SAMADHI. A state of attainment where upon one is in union with oneself; when meditator, object of meditation and meditation are one.

SAMSKARAS. Impressions or imprints on the subconscious mind.

SAMKHYA. Spiritual path, investigating understanding of the existence of the world.

SAMPRAJNATA SAMADHI. The inspired accompaniments of the state of, the fusion of subject and object.

SANATANA DHARMA. Eternal teaching or religion or everlasting path.

SANDHYA BHASA. Twilight language which indicate the way to the Lord.

SASTRA. A sacred text or teaching.

SATCHITANANDA. Absolute existence, consciousness, bliss; perfect love, omniscience, omnipotence, the pure consciousness of all existence.

SATORI. A state of consciousness akin to samadhi; a void; an emptiness full of consciousness.

SATYA. "Truthfulness".

SIDDHAS. "Perfected one;" a person of great spiritual attainment.

SIDDHIS. Accomplishment of supernormal powers.

SIVA. Supreme God which abides in everyone and everything and yet is One above all.

SIVA SHAKTI. The possessor of power; just as the moon does not shine without moonlight, so also siva does not shine without the principle of shakti.

SUTRAS. "Thread;" verses filled with profound knowledge on yoga, law, spiritual wisdom, grammar, medicine, often recited.

T

TANTRA. Scripture which provide detailed instructions on all aspects of religion, science and mysticism.

TAPAS. Severe austerities of a transformative nature, intense practice of Yoga.

TATTVAS. The principles, elements or categories of existence; Sankhya system includes 25.

TYAGA. Detachment from the fruits of one's actions.

U

UPANISHADS. "To sit with one's teacher;" ancient Knowledge past down from guru to disciple; 200 philosophical commentaries on the *Vedas*.

V

VAIRAGYA. Dispassion.

VASAL. "Threshold;" the human body as the container of the Lord.

VEDAS. "Wisdom;" ancient scriptures, which revealed great authority.

VETAVELI. Infinite space.

VIDEHA-MUKTI. "Disemembodied liberation;" liberation at the point of death, when one realizes the self.

APPENDIX A

INDEX OF RED AND PINK LETTER SAYINGS

FROM THE JESUS SEMINAR

(The Five Gospels, pages 549-553)

Title	Av.	Rank	Color
1. Other cheek (Q)			
Matt 5:39	.92	1	Red
Luke 6:29a	.92	1	Red
2. Coat & Shirt (Q)			
Matt 5:40	.92	1	Red
Luke 6:29b	.90	3	Red
3. Congratulations, poor! (Q, Thomas)			
Luke 6:20	.91	2	Red
Thomas 54	.90	3	Red
Matt 5:3	.63	22	Pink
4. Second mile (Q)			
Matt 5:41	.90	3	Red
5. Love of enemies (Q)			
Luke 6:27b	.84	4	Red
Matt 5:44b	.77	9	Red
Luke 6:32, 35a	.56	29	Pink

Title	Av.	Rank	Color
6. Leaven (Q, Thomas)			
Luke 13:20-21	.83	5	Red
Matt 13:33	.83	5	Red
Thom 96:1-2	.65	20	Pink
7. Emperor & God (Thomas, Mark			
Thom 100:2b	.82	6	Red
Mark 12:17b	.82	6	Red
Luke 20:25b	.82	6	Red
Matt 22:21c	.82	6	Red
8. Give to beggars (Q)			
Matt 5:42a	.81	7	Red
Luke 6:30a	.81	7	Red
9. The Samaritan (L)			
Luke 10:30-35	.81	7	Red
10. Congratulations, hungry! (Q, Thomas)			
Luke 6:21a	.79	7	Red
Matt 5:6	.59	26	Red
Thom 69:2	.53	32	Pink
11. Congratulations, sad! (Q)			
Luke 6:21b	.79	8	Red
Matt 5:4	.73	13	Pink
12. Shrewd manager (L)			
Luke 16:1-8a	.77	9	Red
13. Vineyard laborers (M)			
Matt 20:1-15	.77	9	Red
14. Abba, Father (Q)			
Luke 11:2b	.77	9	Red
Matt 6:9b	.77	9	Red

Title	Av.	Rank	Color
Matt 6:9c	.17	68	Black

15. Mustard Seed (Thomas, Mark, Q)

Thom 20:2-4	.76	10	Red
Mark 4:30-32	.74	12	Pink
Luke 13:18-19	.69	17	Pink
Matt 13:31-32	.67	19	Pink

16. On anxieties: don't fret (Thomas, Q)

Thom 36:1	.75	11	Pink
Luke 12:22-23	.75	11	Pink
Matt 6:25	.75	11	Pink

17. Lost Coin (L)

Luke 15:8-9	.75	11	Pink

18. Foxes have dens (Q, Thomas)

Luke 9:58	.74	12	Pink
Matt 8:20	.74	12	Pink
Thom 86:1-2	.67	19	Pink

19. No respect at home (Thomas, John, Mark)

Thom 31:1	.74	12	Pink
Luke 4:24	.71	15	Pink
John 4:44	.67	19	Pink
Matt 13:57	.60	25	Pink
Mark 6:4	.58	27	Pink

20. Friend at midnight (L)

Luke 11:5-8	.72	14	Pink

21. Two masters (Q, Thomas)

Luke 16:13a	.72	14	Pink
Matt 6:24a	.72	14	Pink
Thom 47:2	.65	20	Pink

APPENDIX A: INDEX OF RED AND PINK LETTER SAYINGS FROM JESUS SEMINAR   209

Title	Av.	Rank	Color
Luke 16:13b	.59	26	Pink
Matt 6:24b	.59	26	Pink
22. Treasure (M, Thomas)			
Matt 13:44	.71	15	Pink
Thom 109:1-3	.54	31	Pink
23. Lost sheep (Q, Thomas)			
Luke 15:4-6	.70	16	Pink
Matt 18:12-13	.67	19	Pink
Matt 15:10-11	.48	37	Gray
24. What goes in (Mark, Thomas)			
Mark 7:14-15	.70	16	Pink
Thom 14:5	.67	19	Pink
Matt 15:10-11	.63	22	Pink
25. Corrupt judge (L)			
Luke 18:2-5	.70	16	Pink
26. Prodigal son (L)			
Luke 15:10-11	.70	16	Pink
27. Leave the dead (Q)			
Matt 8:22	.70	16	Pink
Luke 9:59-60	.69	17	Pink
28. Castration for Heaven (M)			
Matt 19:12a	.70	16	Pink
29. By their fruit (Q, Thomas)			
Matt 7:16b	.69	17	Pink
Thom 45.1a	.69	17	Pink
Luke 44b	.56	29	Pink
Matt 12:33a	.44	41	Gray
Matt 7:17-18	.44	41	Gray

Title	Av.	Rank	Color
Luke 6:43	.44	41	Gray
Matt 7:20	.33	52	Gray
Matt 12:33b	.33	52	Gray
Matt 7:16a	.33	52	Gray
Luke 6:44a	.33	52	Gray
Luke 6:46a	.33	52	Gray
Luke 6:45a	.31	54	Gray
Matt 12:35	.31	54	Gray
Thom 45:2-3	.31	54	Gray
Thom 45:1b	.26	59	Gray
Thom 45.4	.24	57	Gray
Matt 12:34	.24	57	Black
Luke 6:45b	.24	57	Black
Matt 7:19	.00	85	Black

30. The dinner party,
    The wedding celebration (Thomas, Q)

Thom 64:1-11	.69	17	Pink
Luke 14:16-23	.56	29	Pink
Matt 22:2-13	.26	59	Gray
Luke 14:24	.00	85	Black
Thom 64:12	.00	85	Black

31. On anxieties, lilies (Q, Thomas)

Luke 12:27-28	.68	18	Pink
Matt 6:28b-30	.68	18	Pink
Thom 36:2	.68	18	Pink

32. Pearl (Thomas, M)

Thom 76:1-2	.68	18	Pink
Matt 13:45-46	.68	18	Pink

Title	Av.	Rank	Color
33. On anxieties, birds (Q)			
Luke 12:24	.67	19	Pink
Matt 6:26	.67	19	Pink
34. Eye of a needle (Mark)			
Matt 19:24	.67	19	Pink
Luke 18:25	.65	20	Pink
Mark 10:25	.64	21	Pink
35. Lord's prayer: revere name (Q)			
Luke 11:2d	.67	19	Pink
Matt 6:9d	.67	19	Pink
36. Lord's prayer:impose rule (Q)			
Luke 11:2e	.67	19	Pink
Matt 6:10a	.58	27	Pink
37. Mountain city (M, Thomas)			
Matt 5:14b	.67	19	Pink
Thomas 32	.54	31	Pink
38. Satan's fall (L)			
Luke 10:18	.67	19	Pink
39. Sly as a snake (M, Thomas)			
Matt 10:16b	.67	19	Pink
Thom 39:3	.65	19	Pink
40. The assassin (Thomas)			
Thom 98:1-3	.65	20	Pink
41. Lend without return (Thomas, Q)			
Thom 95:1-2	.65	20	Pink
Matt 5:42b	.51	34	Pink
Luke 6:34	.44	41	Gray
Luke 6:35c	.27	58	Gray

Title	Av.	Rank	Color
42. Demons by the finger of God (by God's spirit) (Q)			
Luke 11:19-20	.64	21	Pink
Matt 12:27-28	.56	29	Pink
43. Placing the lamp, Lamp & bushel (Q, Mark, Thomas)			
Luke 8:16	.63	22	Pink
Luke 11:33	.63	22	Pink
Mark 4:21	.63	22	Pink
Matt 5:15	.63	22	Pink
Thom 33:2-3	.63	22	Pink
44. Seed & harvest (Mark, Thomas)			
Mark 4:26-29	.63	22	Pink
Thom 21:9	.46	39	Gray
45. Unforgiving slave (M)			
Matt 18:23-34	.63	22	Pink
46. On anxieties: clothing (Q)			
Matt 6:28a	.62	23	Pink
47. Scholars' privileges (Q, Mark)			
Luke 20:46	.61	24	Pink
Mark 12:38-39	.61	24	Pink
Matt 23:5-7	.53	32	Pink
Luke 11:43	.53	32	Pink
48. The leased vineyard (Q, Mark)			
Thom 65:1-7	.61	24	Pink
Thomas 66	.00	85	Black
Mark 12:1-8	.27	58	Gray
Mark 12:9-11	.00	85	Black
Matt 21:33-39	.27	58	Gray
Matt 21:40-43	.00	85	Black

APPENDIX A: INDEX OF RED AND PINK LETTER SAYINGS FROM JESUS SEMINAR

Title	Av.	Rank	Color
Luke 20:9-15a	.27	58	Gray
Luke 20:15b-18	.00	85	Black

49. Left & right hands (M,Thomas)

Matt 6:3	.60	25	Pink
Thom 62:2	.60	25	Pink

50. Sliver & timber (Thomas, Q)

Thom 26:1-2	.60	25	Pink
Matt 7:3-5	.56	29	Pink
Luke 6:41-42	.54	31	Pink

51. True relatives, (Mark, Thomas)

Matt 12:48-50	.60	25	Pink
Thom 99:2	.52	33	Pink
Luke 8:21	.50	35	Gray
Mark 3:33-35	.43	42	Gray
Thom 99:3	.27	58	Gray

52. Lord's prayer: bread (Q)

Matt 6:11	.60	25	Pink
Luke 11:3	.35	50	Gray

53. God & sparrows (Q)

Luke 12:6-7	.60	25	Pink
Matt 10:29-31	.56	9	Pink
Luke 21:18	.27	58	Gray

54. Rich farmer, Rich investor (Thomas, L)

Thom 63:1-6	.60	25	Pink
Luke 12:16-20	.59	26	Pink

55. Money in trust (Q)

Luke 19:13, 15-24	.59	26	Pink
Matt 25:14-28	.59	26	Pink

Title	Av.	Rank	Color
56. Coming of God's imperial rule (Thomas, Q)			
Thom 113:2-4	.59	26	Pink
Luke 17:20-21	.57	28	Pink
Thom 51:2	.00	85	Black
57. Good gifts, (Q)			
Matt 7:9-11	.59	26	Pink
Luke 11:11-13	.43	42	Gray
58. Powerful man (Mark, Q, Thomas)			
Mark 3:27	.59	26	Pink
Matt 12:29	.59	26	Pink
Thom 35:1-2	.59	26	Pink
Luke 11:21-22	.00	85	Gray
59. First & last (Q, Thomas, Mark)			
Matt 20:16	.58	26	Pink
Mark 10:31	.50	35	Gray
Matt 19:30	.50	35	Gray
Luke 13:30	.47	38	Gray
Thom 4:2	.45	40	Gray
Thom 4.3	.00	85	Black
60. Salting the salt (Mark, Q)			
Mark 9:50a	.58	27	Pink
Luke 14:34-35a	.58	27	Pink
Matt 5:13b	.53	32	Pink
61. Pharisee & toll collector (L)			
Luke 18:10-14a	.58	27	Pink
62. Lord's prayer: debts (Q)			
Matt 6;12a	.58	27	Pink
Luke 11:4a-b	.58	27	Gray

APPENDIX A: INDEX OF RED AND PINK LETTER SAYINGS FROM JESUS SEMINAR

Title	Av.	Rank	Color
63. Forgiveness for forgiveness (Mark)			
Luke 6:37c	.57	28	Pink
Mark 11:25	.50	35	Gray
Matt 6:14-15	.45	40	Gray
64. Satan divided (Q, Mark)			
Luke 11:17-18	.57	28	Pink
Matt 12:25-26	.50	35	Gray
Mark 3:23-26	.44	41	Gray
65. Hidden & revealed, Veiled & unveiled (Thomas, Q, Mark)			
Thom 5.2	.57	28	Pink
Thom 6:5	.55	30	Pink
Luke 12:2	.55	30	Pink
Matt 10:26b	.54	31	Pink
Luke 8:17	.54	31	Pink
Thom 6:6	.50	35	Gray
Mark 4:22	.38	47	Gray
Thom 5:3 (Greek)	.00	85	Black
Thom 6:4	.00	85	Black
Matt 10:26a	.00	85	Black
66. Inside & outside (Thomas, Q)			
Thom 89:1-2	.57	28	Pink
Matt 23:25-26	.35	50	Gray
Luke 11:39-41	.32	53	Gray
67. Fasting and wedding (Mark, Thomas)			
Mark 2:19	.56	29	Pink
Matt 9:15a	.56	29	Pink
Luke 5:34	.56	29	Pink
Thom 104:2	.16	69	Black

Title	Av.	Rank	Color
Thom 104:3	.13	72	Black
Luke 5:35	.04	81	Black
Mark 2.20	.04	81	Black
Matt 9:15b	.04	81	Black

68. Better than sinner: love (Q)

Luke 6:32	.56	29	Pink
Matt 5:46	.53	32	Pink

69. Hating one's family (Q, Thomas)

Luke 14:26	.56	29	Pink
Thom 55:1-2a	.49	36	Gray
Matt 10:37	.39	46	Gray
Thom 101:1-3	.20	65	Black

70. Narrow door (Q)

Luke 13:24	.56	29	Pink
Matt 7:13-14	.37	48	Gray

71. Lord of the Sabbath (Mark)

Mark 2:27-28	.56	29	Pink
Matt 12:8	.37	48	Gray
Luke 6:5	.37	48	Gray

72. Difficult with money (Mark)

Mark 10:23	.55	30	Pink
Luke 18:24	.52	33	Pink
Matt 19:23	.51	34	Pink

73. Barren tree (L)

Luke 13:6-9	.54	31	Pink

74. Sower (Mark, Thomas)

Mark 4:3-8	.54	31	Pink
Matt 13:3-8	.53	32	Pink

Title	Av.	Rank	Color
Thom 9:1-5	.52	33	Pink
Luke 8:5-8a	.50	35	Pink
75. On anxieties: one hour (Q)			
Luke 12:25	.54	31	Pink
Matt 6:27	.54	31	Pink
76. Before the judge (Q)			
Luke 12:58-59	.53	32	Pink
Matt 5:25-28	.42	33	Pink
77. Empty jar (Thomas)			
Thom 97:1-4	.53	32	Pink
78. Better than sinners: sunrise (Q)			
Matt 5:45b	.53	32	Pink
79. Into the wilderness (Q, Thomas)			
Matt 11:7-8	.52	33	Pink
Thom 78:1-2	.51	34	Pink
Luke 7:24-25	.50	35	Pink
Thom 78:3	.32	53	Gray
80. Wineskins (Thom, Mark)			
Thom 47:4	.52	33	Pink
Luke 5:37-38	.52	33	Pink
Mark 2:22	.52	33	Pink
Matt 9:17	.49	36	Gray
81. Instructions for the road house (Q)			
Luke 10:7a	.52	33	Pink
82. Children in God's domain (Mark, Thomas)			
Mark 10:14b	.52	33	Pink
Matt 19:14	.52	33	Pink
Luke 18:16	.52	33	Pink

Title	Av.	Rank	Color
83. Return of evil spirits (Q)			
Luke 11:24-26	.52	33	Pink
Matt 12:43-45	.43	42	Gray
84. Fire on earth, (Thomas, Q)			
Thom 10	.52	33	Pink
Luke 12:49	.36	49	Gray
85. Saving one's life (Q, Mark, John)			
Luke 17:33	.52	33	Pink
Matt 16:25	.39	46	Gray
Matt 10:39	.39	46	Gray
Luke 9:24	.39	46	Gray
John 12:25	.30	55	Gray
Mark 8:35	.24	61	Black
86. Ask, seek, knock (Q, Thomas)			
Matt 7:7-8	.51	34	Pink
Luke 11:9-11	.51	34	Pink
Thom 94:1-2	.51	34	Pink
Thom 2:1	.51	34	Pink
Thom 2:2-4	.00	85	Black
87. Aged wine (L, Thomas)			
Luke 5:39	.51	34	Pink
Thom 47:3	.51	34	Pink
Luke 5:39b	.23	62	Black
88. Able-bodied & sick (Gospel fragment 1224, Mark)			
Gospel Fr. 1224 5:2	.51	34	Pink
Matt 9:12	.51	34	Pink
Mark 2:17a	.51	34	Pink
Luke 5:31	.51	34	Pink

Title	Av.	Rank	Color
89. Have & have not (Thomas, Mark, Q)			
Thom 41:1-2	.51	34	Pink
Mark 4:25	.51	34	Pink
Luke 8:18b	.51	34	Pink
Matt 25:29	.49	36	Gray
Matt 13:12	.49	36	Gray
Luke 19:26	.49	36	Gray
90. Instructions for the road: eat (Thomas, Q)			
Thom 14:4a	.51	34	Pink
Luke 10:8	.51	34	Pink
91. Become passersby (Thomas)			
Thomas 42	.50	35	Gray

For information on Babaji's Kriya Yoga please contact:

Babaji's Kriya Yoga and Publications, Inc.
196 Mountain Road · P.O. Box 90
Eastman, Quebec · Canada J0E 1P0
Tel: +1(888) 252-9642 · +1(450) 297-0258 · Fax: +1(450) 297-3957
www.babaji.ca · info@babaji.ca

The Grace of Babaji's Kriya Yoga

A Course of Lessons

An Invitation from Babaji's Kriya Yoga and Publications, Inc.

Two years of Self- Exploration & Discovery

"To hope for a change in human life without a change in human nature is an irrational & un-spiritual proposition; it is to ask for something unnatural & unreal, an impossible miracle." Sri Aurobindo

In our pursuit of our Divine Self we must seek for change in our human nature. But rather than trying to change our nature, we more often merely attempt to reconcile our habits of desire, aversion and fear. So dark elements along with light continue to seek manifestation and arise in the context of our life.

The Grace Course provokes us to delve into our desires, aversions and fears in order to reveal to us our truth and falseness.

As ingrained habits and instincts are probed, weaknesses will be amplified. This process is personal and profound and real work.

Have You Sincerely and Genuinely Considered:

- How far can discipline and personal effort get you?
- What is Grace and is it absolutely necessary for Self-Knowledge?
- Is your Ego really so bad?
- Must I love everyone, or just do my duty?
- How can I keep love from diminishing into attachment or dissolving into anger or indifference?
- Why is life so full of desire, aversion and fear?
- Is there ever a need for fear?
- How can I learn to use my willpower effectively to overcome my resistances?
- Is there a Higher Will for my life, and if so, how can I learn to connect with it?
- Is what you can "see," even in meditation, ever the true Self?

The entire course consists of 24 monthly lessons. Each lesson is about 15 pages. You may subscribe one year at a time: $108 per year

To subscribe to this course, contact us at: **Babaji's Kriya Yoga Publications**

196 Mountain Road · PO Box 90 · Eastman · QC · J0E 1P0 Canada · **www.babaji.ca**

THE VOICE OF BABAJI
A TRILOGY ON KRIYA YOGA

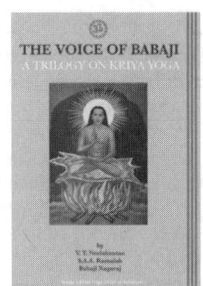

Sri V.T. Neelakantan recorded verbatim a series of talks given by Satguru Kriya Babaji in 1953. These are a fountain of delight and inspiration, illuminating the Kriya Yoga path towards God realization, unity in diversity and universal love. They also reveal the magnetic personality of Babaji and how he supports us all, with much humour and wisdom. 216 pages, 4 maps, Includes the fascinating accounts of the meetings with Babaji in Madras and in the Himalayas by authors V.T. Neelakantan and Yogi S.A.A. Ramaiah. Out of print for nearly 50 years, they are profound and important statements from one of the world's greatest living spiritual masters. 8 pages in color. 534 pages. ISBN 978-1-895383-23-2. Canada: CAD$41.49, USA: US$31.50, Asia & Europe: US$50.50

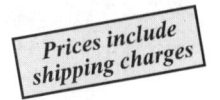

Prices include shipping charges

THIRUMANDIRAM:
A Classic of Yoga and Tantra
by Siddhar Thirumoolar

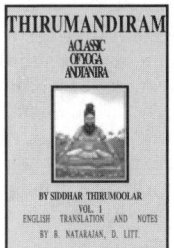

Edited by M. Govindan. Get connected to the roots of Yoga with the first English translation of Thirumoolar's classic masterpiece of Yoga, tantra, and Saiva Siddhantha, the gospel of the Tamil Yoga Siddhas. "The Thirumandiram is as important as the *Bhagavad Gita, The Sutras of Patanjali* and *Yoga Vasistha*...". This outstanding text is now available in a fine 3-volume edition, thanks to Marshall Govindan's labor of love" - Georg Feuerstein, Ph.D., contributing editor of *Yoga Journal*. 3,047 gem-like verses, with introduction, explanatory notes, index, glossary, illustrations. 828 pages in 3 volumes, 6" x 9". ISBN 978-1-895383-02-7. Canada: CAD$56.86, USA: US$44.25, Asia & Europe: US$76.75

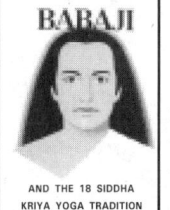

BABAJI AND THE 18 SIDDHA KRIYA YOGA TRADITION
8th edition
by M. Govindan

A rare account of Babaji, the Himalayan master who developed Kriya Yoga, the Siddhas, his source of inspiration and the principles of Kriya Yoga. Guidelines for its practice. 216 pages, 4 maps, 33 color photos, 100 bibliographic references and glossary. 6" x 9". ISBN 978-1-895383-00-3. Canada: CAD$31.08, USA: US$24.45, Asia & Europe: US$32.45

THE YOGA OF SIDDHA BOGANATHAR
by T.N. Ganapathy, P.h.D

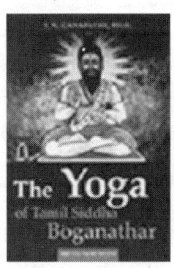

Boganathar was the guru of Kriya Babaji Nagaraj. Boganathar lived an extremely long life through the use of alchemy and special breathing techniques. He traveled all over the world and provided his disciples an illumined path to Self-realization and integral transformation of human nature into divinity. His astounding life provides a shining example of our human potential. The present work provides a biography of Boganathar, and **a translation and commentary of many of his poems.** ISBN 978-1-895383-19-5 **Vol. 1** Canada: CAD$32.88, USA: US$24.95, Asia & Europe: US$43.95. ISBN 978-1-895383-26-3 **Vol. 2** Canada: CAD$37.78, USA: US$28.45, Asia & Europe: US$60.95

Other titles available from Kriya Yoga Publications, Inc.:

KRIYA YOGA SUTRAS OF PATANJALI AND THE SIDDHAS
by Marshall Govindan

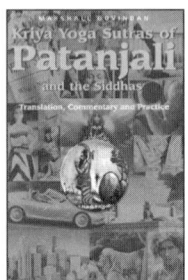

This translation is both easy to understand and precise. The commentary reveals for the first time the closeness of Patanjali to the Tamil Siddha philosophical tradition. A unique commentary which provides for each verse "practices" or Kriyas useful for the Kriya Yoga initiate and non-initiate alike. **"Indispensable for students of Kriya Yoga... a valuable addition to the study of Yoga in general and the Yoga-Sutra in particular. I can wholeheartedly recommend it." From the foreword by** Georg Feuerstein, Ph D. **"An excellent and easily readable commentary"** - David Frawley. **"A significant contribution to the sadhana of every serious yoga student"** - Yoga Journal. 220 pages, Sanskrit transliteration, indexes of Sanskrit and English terms, index of Kriyas indicated in the verses. ISBN 978-1-895383-12-6. Canada: CAD$34.60, USA: US$25.50, Asia & Europe: US$44.50

BABAJI'S KRIYA HATHA YOGA SELF-REALIZATION THROUGH ACTION WITH AWARENESS
DVD
With Marshall Govindan & Durga Ahlund

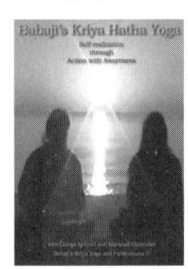

Learn the 18 postures developed by Babaji Nagaraj and become the Seer, not the Seen! Become aware of what is aware! Bliss arises! This unique, beautiful, 2 hour video provides careful detailed instructions in not only the technical performance of each posture, but also in the higher states of consciousness which they awaken. Make your practice of yoga deeply meditative. Taught in progressive stages with preparatory variations making them accessible to the beginner and challenging for the experienced student of Yoga."**Earnest, unique and inspiring**" - Yoga Journal. ISBN 978-1-895383-18-8. Canada: CAD$24.14, Quebec: CN$26.73, USA: US$23.94, Asia & Europe: US$26.45

THE YOGA OF THE 18 SIDDHAS: An Anthology
Edited by T.N. Ganapathy

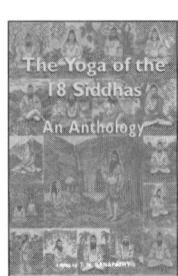

The Yoga of the Eighteen Siddhas: An Anthology includes a biography, an English translation and commentary of selected poems for each of the 18 Siddhas. It contains not only revolutionary statements of those great men and women who have reached the furthest heights of human potential, but also serves as a roadmap for the rest of us to follow. The Siddhas who represent the best of what we can all aspire to become have given us illuminated writings, so filled with the light of God realization that they can have an impact on our heart and mind, just by studying them. This book takes us along a path of Jnana Yoga. 642 pages. ISBN 978-1-895383-24-9. Canada: CAD$40.43, USA: US$30.45, Asia & Europe: US$62.95

To order our publications or tapes:

Call toll free: 1-888-252-9642 or (450) 297-0258, Fax: (450) 297-3957, E-mail: info@babaji.ca

You may have your order charged to a VISA/MasterCard/AmericanExpress or send a cheque or International money order to:

Kriya Yoga Publications, P.O. Box 90, Eastman, Quebec, Canada, J0E 1P0

All prices include postal shipping charges and taxes.
or place your order securely via our E-commerce at www.babaji.ca